Mindful

Messages

Healing Thoughts for the Hip and Hop Descendants from the Motherland

Deborah Day

Ashay by the Bay   **Union City, California**

Publisher: Ashay by the Bay
          Union City, California
          www.ashaybythebay.com

Editor: L. Kahlil Patterson
        A4know Enterprise

Book Cover Design by Deborah Day

Book Cover Design Art and Art Illustrations by Adrienne Drayton

Library of Congress Card Number 2004090000

ISBN 0970404824

Printed in the United States of America

First to the Divine Creator with whom I am one.
Then to my ancestors who are many and awake.
And to all the young and old Hip Hop
descendants from the Motherland.

Acknowledgments

My first acknowledgment goes to the Divine Creator, to whom I give praise every day for my blessings. I also give thanks to my ancestors (thank you Grand Daddy) and my parents John and Katie Windley Day who first instilled in their children God's love and a sense of their own potential.

Much love and thanks to my son Hilton Jamal, for his love and inspiration, patience and understanding. I would also like to thank my brothers and sisters and their families for their encouragement. Sincere thanks also to one of my teachers and dear sista friends, Selena Awolley and brother Bart Elliot for their friendship, knowledge and wisdom.

Many thanks and recognition to L. Kahlil Patterson for his generous spirit, refined editing and post development strategies. A blessed thank you to Adrienne Drayton for her beautiful art illustrations and trusting spirit. Also, I would like to acknowledge and thank Dr. Kwaku Ofori Ansa of Howard University, an Adinkra scholar for allowing me to use his designs and research in this book. Special thanks and appreciation to the following people: Maurice Graham for his forward thinking; Dr. Robert Scott for his sincere dedication; Letitia Burton for her warm spirit and life-skills knowledge; Dr. Stephen Lee for his medical expertise; Joy Tang for her vision of healing; Mosi Michael A. Buck for his friendship and insight on HIV/AIDS; Jim Taylor for his expert research; George Jackson for his suggestions and Mr. B. for being there. Also I am grateful to all of my "sista" and "brotha" friends for their encouragement during the completion of this book.

Lastly, my deepest thanks to all the members of the Alameda County African American State of Emergency HIV/AIDS Task Force, in Oakland and the staff at the Ella Hill Hutch Community Center in San Francisco for believing in my book and my mentoring program. Also I must thank the young people who participated in my first teen forum and the many promising students I have come to know.

CONTENTS

Acknowledgments
Forward

Introduction/Instructions 1

Mindfulness Manifests Miracles 7

Part One: The Poetry 13

Part Two: Akoben 51
   Drugs Definitely Don't Do
   Special Message for the Hip
   Special Message for the Hop
   Living Life with HIV/AIDS
   10 Ways the Mindful Messenger Can Help Heal the World
   Real Facts About HIV/AIDS and African Americans

Part Three: The Agreements 113
   Mindfulness Meditation

Part Four: The Adinkra Symbols 121
   Origins and Meaning
   Health Alert: Tattoos and Body Piercing

Part Five: HIV/AIDS Nationwide Listing 137

Bibliography 171
About the Author 175
Mindful Notes 176

FORWARD

Living with HIV since 1983 has taught me a few things about life because I now realize, the thoughts I think about myself directly affect my health and well being. My childhood and young adult years were filled with violence, neglect, alienation and addiction. I inherited my parent's addiction to alcohol and co-dependency and covered my pain with drugs, sex, anger and money. It was this frame of mind that caused me to engage in careless, indiscriminate sexual behavior, which is how I contracted the HIV virus.

In 1996, I founded a non-profit organization called AID for AIDS Africa, responding to the AIDS epidemic and the underlying perception of abuse. Our purpose is to use education and medical intervention as tools to over come the issue of fear and denial as it exist in the African American and African communities. Since 1998 I have traveled to Africa ten times speaking my truth and envisioning my way out of sickness, lack and limitation. In my travels, I witnessed a lot of pain and suffering which was brought on by AIDS. This devastating reality, made me realize the importance of connecting African communities in the U.S. to African communities in the Motherland because not only do we share the same ancestors, but those of us living with HIV/AIDS also share a common desire to live with dignity.

Since my recovery from 27 years of substance abuse, I have come to love myself unconditionally. My healing began the moment I changed the message in my head. I now see new possibilities for living and I have found new meaning in life. MINDFUL MESSAGES is a giant step in the direction of awareness. MINDFUL MESSAGES teaches us to be "mindful" of our thoughts and feeling, for "we become as we believe." I hold this book out to you as one possible way to "keep the high watch" for signs of change for the better.

Maurice Graham, President and Founder AID for AIDS/Africa

Introduction / Instructions

Mindful Messages *Healing Thoughts for the Hip and the Hop Descendants from the Motherland,* is a collection of healing thoughts that were sent to me from Divine Spirit. I feel blessed in sharing them with you and I hope others will find a special message or messages that resonates with their spirit.

This book is intended for everyone, but it is particularly for African American youngsters of the Hip Hop generation. However, if Africa is the Motherland and the origin of all civilizations, then is not everyone, as the subtitle suggests a "Descendant of the Motherland?" And are we not in truth all Africans? And does the older generation still think they are the hippest and does not the younger generation think it's got all the Hop? And what has all this got to do with Hip Hop, other than the fact that Hip Hop's origins and "beats" are rooted in the oral tradition of our great ancestors.

The fact is we both (the Hip and the Hop the young and the old) have a collective and genetic history that binds all of us to the Motherland. As a race of people we shall acknowledge that bond and our oneness with our brothers and sisters in Africa. We also need to be mindful of the universal truth, "What happens to one happens to the other." But for all practical purposes I am referencing African Americans when I refer to the black community in America, even though in my heart and soul I know we are all Africans. So when your souls looks back (*Sankofa*), listen up and be still you might learn something new! By the way did you know that the word for Hip Hop in South Africa is "*Kwaito*" which means clever tongue?

My relationship with Hip Hop is not extensive, but it does go back a few years. When rap first began I was in my twenties, living in

Chicago dancing to the music of Run DMC and Kool Moe Dee. Now I am in my forties and living in California and listening to TuPac, Public Enemy, Mos Def, NAS, 50 Cent, Common and some of the other popular rappers. Even though I have a great appreciation for jazz, blues, gospel and some rock and roll, I like a little Hip Hop too.

Hip Hop is the dominant youth culture and it is powerful because many young people around the world identify with its urban energy. It was created from within by talented young brothers and sisters in the "hood" who were speaking their truth in rhythms and rhymes, "to being Black in America." This spiritual yet volatile energy engulfed everything real and personal in its path including music, dance, language and fashion, forming a life-style that evolved into its own culture. Except for the glorification of violence, sex and drugs and the degrading lyrics and images of women, the music of Hip Hop has many redeeming qualities. And like spoken word it can be used to entertain, empower and educate.

Moving to California proved to be very challenging. Meditation and writing helped me to stay focused and balanced. After a few life altering moments and a vision, God started pointing me in a different direction. I had already invested hundreds of hours of research in another subject, but I had to lay it aside. What emerged was a book of poetry that also focused on the HIV/AIDS (human immunodeficiency virus and acquired immuno deficiency syndrome) epidemic that is plaguing the continent of Africa and the African American community.

I really became concerned about the HIV/AIDS epidemic when I learned African Americans were leading the United States HIV population trends, and that the lethal virus was spreading faster among us than any other ethnic group. Even though I had been watching the path of the disease for a number of years, it never occurred to me that African Americans would soon account for over 50% of the newly reported HIV cases. Nor did I foresee the certain genocide of millions of newly freed South Africans being annihilated by this disease. Admittedly, I am skeptical of some of the statistics and the social political issues surrounding the epidemic. However, now that HIV/ AIDS is a global pandemic that is a threat to everyone's health and many third world economies, I believe there is only time to look inward and push outward toward "mindful intervention" and prepare our young people for the future.

This book contains five parts and is designed as an educational and motivational tool that can be used by parents, educators, mentors and young people to learn more about African and African American culture and HIV/AIDS Awareness and Prevention. It begins with a definition and overview of Mindfulness that also includes simple instructions to guide one through a Mindful Meditation. Then it moves into the "creative healing consciousness of poetry." After reading this book, one should be able to recognize and understand the cause of HIV/AIDS so they will know how to best prevent this disease and help others.

Part One has 26 poems, one for each letter of the alphabet that touches on the epidemic or identifies some other socioeconomic political issue. The first poem is titled "Attention." It's message promotes abstinence as the best preventive solution to stop the spread of AIDS and it reminds us that the ancestors are awake and anticipating our accountability. My poems are written in an assonance and alliteration style and they flow with some of the consciousness of Hip Hop. They are filled with insight, motherly advice and spiritual truths. Also in Part One you will find soulful black and white images by reknown artist Adrienne Drayton that are sure to lock one into a "memorable mindful meditation."

Part Two of the book is titled, "Akoben," it is an Adinkra word that means a "call to action." It deals specifically with the HIV/ AIDS epidemic and points to the serious need for all African Americans to look at how the disease is socially and culturally impacting our families and communities. In this section I highlight statistics on various populations according to the Centers for Disease Control (CDC), the government agency that monitors disease trends and sets policy for local and state CDC supported agencies. I also give suggestions on what everyone can do collectively and individually to stop the spread of HIV and join in the healing of the community. Even though the HIV/AIDS messages are for everyone, I included special messages for two important groups. They are whom I refer as the "Hip" (parents/educators and mentors) and the "Hop" (sexually active and or non-active teens) who may or may not be "at risk." In this section the facts on STD's HIV transmission, drugs, abstinence, safe sex and "at risk" behaviors and relationships are vitally important, because the disease is reportedly spreading faster among African American young people ages (13-19) then any other ethnic youth population.

In this section, also one will find insightful African proverbs among the text. And you will read about the growing trend among many enlightened teens to "wait on sex." I am promoting abstinence first and reminding our young people that if they are already sexually active to practice safe sex. In addition to the aforementioned key points, are several personal stories of African and African Americans who are living with HIV/AIDS, which hopefully will bring more compassion for those afflicted and affected by the disease.

✳✳✳ **Part Three** contains a letter to parents and adolescent/teens reminding them of the need to schedule some quality time to discuss some of the issues (sex and drugs) that cause HIV/AIDS and other STD's. (As the experts say, if you want to protect your children ask a lot of questions and get to know their friends.) I am also urging parents to encourage their son or daughter to get tested if they think they may have participated in any high-risk sexual activity. This part of the book also contains two agreements, the "My Choice to Abstain from Sex Agreement" and the "My Choice to Stay Drug Free Agreement." The agreements are designed to help young people set goals and take steps towards achieving their own personal empowerment.

Part Four describes and illuminates the Adinkra symbols. It also provides information on the West African symbols origin and history. I included them because they are powerful spiritual connectors to our ancestors and many young people are identifying with their traditional cultural symbols when getting tattooed and body piercings. However, they are not always aware that they can get infected with HIV or another STD through contaminated needles.

Part Five is a nationwide resource listing that contains over 700 HIV/AIDS agencies, clinics, organizations and websites. They can be contacted for HIV/AIDS education and prevention and other HIV/AIDS related services.

In conclusion, I would like to say something profound and memorable but all I could come up with is this. Our minds are bombarded with messages 24/7/365. We receive ongoing messages from "Divine Spirit", our ancestors, parents, family, friends and neighbors, the government, the church, the media, society-at-large and also in our dreams. Some messages are positive and others are negative. Some are clear others are subliminal (hidden). Together they form our values, beliefs, behaviors, judgments and opinions, which ultimately influences our conscious mind, our character and our choices.

Just remember, the key to understanding the real meaning of any message is to first know thyself, (*Nsoroma*)– you are a spiritual being and a Divine child of god). Secondly, know your tribal self, (*Sankofa* – know your origins, your ancestors and your true history) and finally seek to know the sender, whoever or whatever it might be. Most importantly be mindful and be encouraged for the journey. *Ashe!*

November 4th Thurs, 2021 @ 7:45am
study materials for my early bible study
meditions. Reference affirmations

∅ Iyanla Vanzant

Daily Meditions for African American
Women

Mindfulness

Christmas gift to
Self

Purchase
Leather
Jesus
Calling

Also   Purple
                                        Study
Jesus Calling for scriptures in Bible

pass on to next person the hardback version

purchase calendar for end of year to

next year Daily Planner.

"Mindfulness Manifests Miracles"

✳ ✳ ✳ ✳ ✳ ✳ ✳ ✳ ✳

There is a lyric by Snoop Dogg where he says "I got my mind on my money and my money on my mind." For the most part he was expressing his conscious concern about his finances. He was also being a bit mindful.

What is Mindfulness

Basically mindfulness is a conscious state of being completely aware and in the present moment. The present moment meaning right here and right now this very breath and moment. It is a subtle process that many probably are not familiar with but do naturally everyday. But what if we could learn more about mindfulness to raise our level of awareness to open the doors to our Creative Spirit to increase our self knowledge and personal power?

Another way to describe mindfulness is as a "knowing attention" to what is going on "inside" your head and not jumping to react to the clusters of thoughts and feelings continuously moving across your mind. This may sound easy to do, but in truth it takes practice. When you are being mindful, your mind is operating from a calm centered state of consciousness that is in a watchful mode not a busy thinking mode.

Mindfulness, synonymous with mindful meditation is a universal human concept that is one of the virtues of Buddhism. Devotees of this popular Eastern religious philosophy have been practicing this form of meditation for over two thousand years. The ancient civilizations of Africa, the worlds first teachers, were aware of the enormous benefits of mindful meditation and practiced it along with prayer. Our ancient ancestors also learned that when combined with discipline, mindful meditation could open doors to creativity that revealed their inner healing and peace.

Mindfulness vs. Consciousness

Light and non-judgmental *involved*

When it comes to the inner workings of the mind one can easily distinguish between mindfulness and consciousness. For instance mindfulness energy is clear, light and detached. Whereas, consciousness energy is laden with mental and emotional attachments. Another noticeable difference is that mindfulness activity is non-judgmental and observant. Consciousness activity, on the other hand is very judgmental and involved. Consciousness in it's simplest form is an internal manifestation of knowledge, but what young people must learn is "self knowledge" so that they can learn who and what they are.

Ancient African Societies and Our Ancestors

The ancient African societies of our ancestors had highly organized social structures. Both concepts, mindfulness and consciousness were integral to their religion, spirituality, rituals, customs and daily life. It was also emphasized during Rites of Passage when the elders imparted important oral ancestral knowledge and wisdom to educate and prepare their youth for adulthood. On those occasions, each boy and girl would be given serious social training that each was expected to learn. While the Elders followed tribal traditions, they invested valuable time and energy teaching the youth self-knowledge and guiding them towards identifying their individual intrinsic gifts and talents.

Every Child is a Treasure

These moral and spiritual instructions were very important as it prepared young people to be wiser adults who would continue to pass this knowledge on to their children. The ancestors believed that every child was a treasure and contributed to the shared vision of the village. And so it was that some youth were born into nobility or special ranking and were placed on thrones (Kings and Queens and leaders), some were identified as future shaman (healers/medical doctors) and others were chosen to be the griots (historians/teachers). The gatherers, herdsman, fishermen or farmers (builders /tradesman) were selected early on too, while others were called to be craftsman, singers, musicians and dancers (artists/entertainers). And a few were called to be fearless warriors (protectors). However, they were all taught that they were children of God and the values of love, respect, trust and honoring and remembering their ancestors and traditions. Of the many survival life skills they passed onto youth were, how to recognize danger, how to protect themselves from predators and how to defend the village if needed. Otherwise, any one of them could meet their fate traveling down the wrong path, unaware of the poisonous snakes and other dangerous creatures awaiting them in the jungle.

Survival of the Village

Mindfulness and consciousness practiced together creates understanding, which leads to wisdom and compassion. In most African villages everyone cooperated and understood that the survival of the village depended upon the survival of the family and the tribe. Members participated in the circle of life by respecting the family, the ancestors and the oneness of Mother Earth and the Divine Creator. Everyone worked collectively together to maintain balance and harmony. In so doing, they also maintained their culture, traditions and history which brought stability and order to the family and the village, ensuring that their way of life was peaceful, productive and prosperous for all.

The Elders

Today it is still important part of African American tradition for young people to respect and listen to their elders because they "hold the knowledge" and they have the life experience. The elders in your community are very aware of the chaos in consciousness that has grown between genders and generations due to drugs, violence, mis-education, lack of values, fast food and other social ills. They are also aware that just as negative behaviors are learned, they can be un-learned with faith, self love and positive behavior. Most of the elders remember or participated in the Civil Rights Movement and they know what it means to be an African American in this country and to have your rights violated. The elders know that the struggle to uplift our people continues and it is urgently necessary that young people "step up" to their responsibility because racism is still very much a reality.

The Power of Mindfulness

Mindful meditation is powerful and life transforming. By being more aware and focused, young people can use their minds to be better disciplined students in and out of the classroom. Enabling them to achieve higher grades, improve sports performance, nurture relationships and to avoid drugs and other bad influences that cause "at risk" behavior. Adults and parents can also benefit from practicing mindfulness by relaxing and releasing daily stress.

Each and every person in both the Hip and the Hop generation should tap into the power of mindfulness and collectively raise their consciousness as we move forward writing our own history and identifying our own problems and solutions. While we mindfully prepare to delete the worry, doubt and fear of any challenging condition including the threat of HIV/AIDS. Let us reclaim our rightful African heritage that the Divine Creator wants us to have. Let us be mindful of the present, while we purposefully seek to learn more about our past, so that we can prepare for the future. Let us proclaim with our ancestors, health, happiness and prosperity as our natural birthright here on this earth.

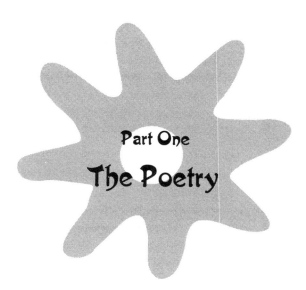

Part One

The Poetry

Attention

All AFRICANS and AFRICANS in AMERICA
Adults & Adolescents.
Akoben!
Announcing AIDS AWARENESS, AIDS ALERT.
Abandon "at risk" active abusive amorous activities and affairs.
Abstract animal amok.
Author's address and apology anonymous.
Atragedy.
An ANNIHILATION!

Anti-discriminatory absolutely attacks all.
Arrogant attitudes aside,
ANCESTORS awake and anticipating accountability.
All Africans ascending ... Amen Ra.
Ancients alternative answer ... ABSTAIN!

Aim at archetype ask advice and acknowledge activities.
Adapt agreement and agenda and adhere.
Adjust associations and affiliations.
Assume appropriate authentic Africentric attitude and actions.
ABSTINENCE answers abortion activists and advocates.

ABSTINENCE anchors Angels amplified attendance and
amazing anointment.
ABSTINENCE affirms admiration and abundance.
Atone Allah alive Amen.

Africans and Africans in America,
Advocate ABSTINENCE and all attention to attendance and
ACADEMIC ACHIEVEMENT.
And always award Africans and Africans in America for our
accomplishments and appreciate our ancestor's ancient arts,
traditions and magnificent contributions.
Ashe!

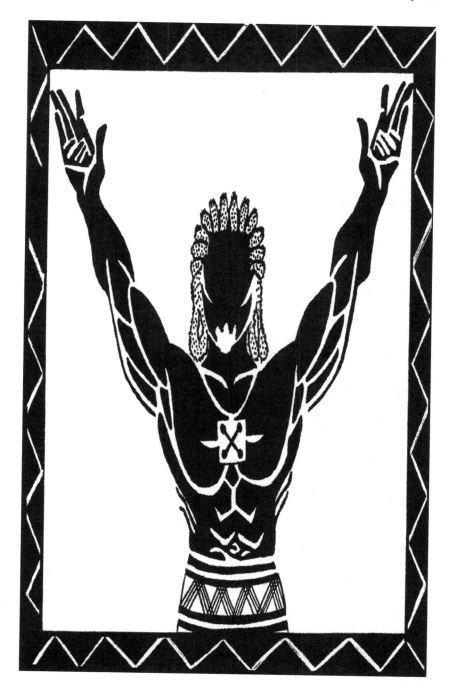

BROTHERS BIRTHRIGHT

BORN believing, BLESSED Bliss.
Baby Buddhas breathing balance, breathing bravery.
Brought over on the boat.
Bred biologically big boned, broad backs, bodies bustin.
Burning hearts beating boldly, because being born black became
"Blackman's Bondage".
Bane supremacist bull!
Brothers were brainwashed!
Brothers were bamboozled!
"BLACK IS BEAUTIFUL", "Black is Brilliant", "Black is the Blueprint".
Brothers beginning, before beyond slavery's blatant interruption.
Brings us back to.

BORN believing, BLESSED Bliss.
Bright, beautiful, blood brothers.
Being becoming one and breaking bread.
Build bigger better BLACK BUSINESSES.
Black entrepreneurs burgeoning power brokers ... Bank.
Build bridges, buy books ... Bank.
Brothers be booking, better yet, Bachelors, Masters, Ph. D's.
Board of Directors, left brain right brain Benjamin Ballers ... Bank.
Bounce balls, big balls!
Brainstorm, break barriers, bring on the beats, blast the bell curve,
B L A C K   P O W E R!

Banish bad burdensome bling blingin behavior: bullets,
bloodshed, blame barking, back biting, back sliding, bigotry,
boredom and bad boys gang banging.
Boooooom!
Behold blind bondage BROTHERS!
BROTHAS bonding brings bounty.
Bottomline Brothers. Be true to Boo and the Babies too.
BELIEVE BE BOLD ... Bravo!

CHERISH CHILDREN'S COSMOS

Create colorful caring COMMUNITIES.
Cerebral "Circle of Life".
Connect, communicate, choose chief, conform covenant, coordinate counsel, contribute clock and colonize.
Collaborate with coalitions and committees, collectively cooperate and cap consumer consumption, CULTIVATE CULTURE, celebrate church and computerize.

CONDEMN CORRUPTION & CONSPIRACIES.
Curse crack and cocaine, cancel crime, conquer condom contraceptive confusion and contracted diseases.
Cut the conflicts.
Counteract crisis.
CLAIM CONTROL!
Cannot compromise community.

Center self.
Celibacy.
Collect clear conscious, chant.
CALL CHARACTER, call courage, call confidence, call commitment.
Call compassion, come correct.
Call civilized clean cut conditions.
Call on the CREATOR, Celestial Clout!

Champion CIVIL RIGHTS.
Classify current events and CHOOSE CORRECT COLLEGE curriculum, careers and compensation ... crash ceilings!
Commanding caviar, cheddar cheese, chitlins and corn bread.
Capitalize.
Challenge Congress, consequences costly.
Conceive corporate corridors and check certified credentials.
C O M MU N I C A T E in the COSMOS.

Drugs

DEFINITELY DON'T DO!
Drugs dropped in the hood delivers DEATH, DIScord, DISrespect, DISease, DISharmony, DIStrust, DIVORCE, DESTRUCTION!
Drugs drags you into the devils dark dungeon.
Drugs in the diaspora damage and demoralize descendants for decades.
 D.O.A. dusted dopes ... drugs dissssssssss!
DRUGS WILL DESTROY YOUR DESTINY.

DEFEAT DANGEROUS DRUG DILEMMA.
Dispose of the crazy drugs and drama.
Decide your dharma.
HIV and other STD's are rooted in irresponsible drug karma.

Discriminate, disarm and distance drug dealers.
Drop desperate dates and dependant druggie doers.
DON'T DRINK and DRIVE.
Don't drown stay alive.

Defy depravity, DIG DEEP and DETOX.
Develope different direction you own the clock.
Delete the data, disengage, deprogram and d e t a c h!
Dominate your daily duties stay strong do not attack.

Don't delay.
Don't disobey.
Define duty and declare DIVINE discipline.
Degrees do matter because the ancestors are listenin.

DEMAND DIGNITY demonstrate diplomacy.
Determine destination, difficult doors do open.
Design dance ... drum diligently.
DISCOVER DEVOTION and d:i:g:/i:t:i:z:e d*r*e*a*m*s.com.

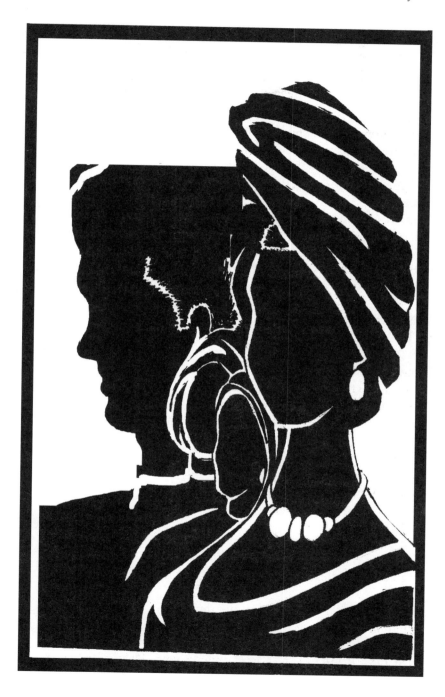

Everyday Escape

EVERYDAY EXCUSE EGO.
Eliminate and exhale empty elements.
Embody eternal essence, essence, essence, essence ... eternity.

ENTERTAIN MINDFULNESS AND ENLIGHTENMENT.
Expand existential environment.
Explore earth and extend existing empire.

EXPECT EXCELLENT EDUCATION.
Exercise effort, equality and elite matriculation.
Examine everything, everything, everything, everything.

Establish ethical employment, e-commerce and e-learning.
ENDORSE ETHNIC ENTERPRISES AND
ENTREPRENEURING.
Equivalent to true ECONOMIC desire.

Encourage enthusiasm and enjoy everlasting dreams.
Exchange energies exponentially and exemplify esteem.
Ebonize, electrify and edify ... Ebonize, electrify and edify.

EMANCIPATE EVERYONE.
Embrace expresso evolution.
Evolve light the fire.

Fathers Forgive

FATHERS FORGIVE.
Forgive fathers.
Face fears.
Forget faults and frontin.
Find faith, forebears found faith.
Fulfill fundamental function, fate.

FAMILY FIRST.
Follow fathers footsteps to fountainhead ... FATHERHOOD.
Form friendships for future.
Find familiar forum and foster feminine support, fellowship.
Focus on fitness.
Fashioning folktails and following feelings for fun ... fraternize.

FORMAT FINANCES.
Figure free enterprise financial foresight.
Feed flock, find a cure and philosophize freely.
Fertilize farm for fresh fruit ... flourish.
Fist fight fair and forget foolish firearms.
Forget fightin ... frightens fragmented families.
Freeze the fog ... fortify the family.

FUNNEL FORTUNES.
Fillup fierce formidable foundations ... life force.
Fly fast forward.
F r u i t i on.
Flow.
Funky like phat full bodied flava!
Finally for the 411.
Finish favorably.
FAMILY FIRST FOREVER FOR FREEDOM!

GOD'S GIFTS

GOD GIVES GIANT GLORIOUS GIFTS.
Genuine genetic genes.
God guides.
Gotta go along to get gleaming goodies.
Generous gentle good God.
Going with God guarantees great gratification.

God isn't gold.
God isn't the government.
GOD GOVERNS.
God isn't genome.
Good gosh almighty, God is the guardian.
GOD is groovy.
God got game.

Get grounded genius.
Get a Guru.
Get goals.
Get good grades!
God forgives.
GRACE GARNERS GROWTH, GET GOD.
Get a grip.

Get grassroots gumption.
Goofy games gotta go.
Gambling, graffiti, greed, guns, gangstas early graves gotta go.
Guilt, gutter gossip, ghetto gimmicks, gender gaps and gettin sexed
without protection, gotta go.
GENERATES HIV/AIDS GLOBAL GENOCIDE GET IT!

Getup great generation graduate.
Get the gift.
Get the Gospel.
GET THE GHOST ... GET GOD.

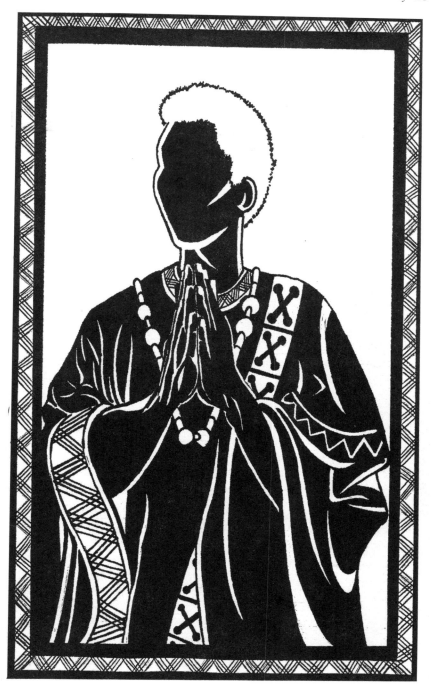

Heroes Heritage

Heroes heritage.
HEIRS ... HEIRESSES.
Hold honest head, heredity ... homage.
Host honorable happy wholistic household.
HIP HOP how handsome.
HA HA HA!
Hallelujah!
HOMEBOY HOMEGIRL HARMONIZING.
Holy Spirit's happenin in the hood.
Habari Gani?
Hotep ... HOLLA!

HASTEN HUMANITY'S HEALING be humble not hypocritical.
Harness, handsome hunks and hotties hard heads, hormones and hedonist habits.
Hush homey, hit a homer.
Hang a hat don't haggle him or her.
Hems in any possible HIV, Herpes and other STD's.
Hug your honey don't lie and hide.
HAVE HEART and HUMOR be smart you must decide.

Heroes history have to have helping hands.
Help HEAL the HUNGRY and the HOMELESS.
He ain't heavy take a stand.
HUMAN HEALTH, haunted by hate, hyped hostility, hollow heedless homicides, homophobia and HIV/AIDS.
Holocaust how horrible but then so was the African slave trade!
Heroes hurt to however heroes have to have higher hopes and higher ideals.

Heroes Harvest Heaven ... Harambee!

I

I,
I am,
IMAGE,
Imagine,
IMAGINATION.

Infinite ideas.
Invisable inheritance ... INTUITION.
Interpretation,
Invest inward ... inside.

Independent I insignificant.
Intellectual ideologies insignificant.
Imperialistic idols and icons insignificant.
Incarnation instills INSTANT IDENTITY INSURANCE.
Intelligence, Imani, Insight, Instinct, Integrity, Inspiration, Illumination,
Increase, Increase, Increase.

Its incomprehensibly intoxicating.
It immortalizes I.

It's your imperative identity.

JOURNEY JOYOUSLY

Jumpin, juba, jiggy, jazzy, jumbo JOY!
Just be aware junior of the streets jousting jones and juggernauts.
JAIL JEOPARDIZES JUBILATION.
Jammin juniors juice and junking juniors reputation.

JADED JUVENILE JUSTICE.
Juniors JUNGLE.
Jeepers no justice for junior.
JUNIOR REALLY IS A GENIUS.

Junior became frustrated, flunked school and tried to keep it clean.
But the streets was his home and just to unforgiving and mean.
Jury and jacked up judicial John Hancock's counted three strikes and
joined jurisdictions.
Jerking juniors chain against his family and his teachers wishes.

JADED JUVENILE JUSTICE.
Juniors JUNGLE.
Jeepers no justice for junior.
JUNIOR REALLY IS A GENIUS.

Judge, Judge, Judge,
Juinior needs a job and mentor not a cold jail cell and a sentence.
Junior justify and jumpstart your journey all over.
JOIN the mighty JAH also know as JEHOVAH.

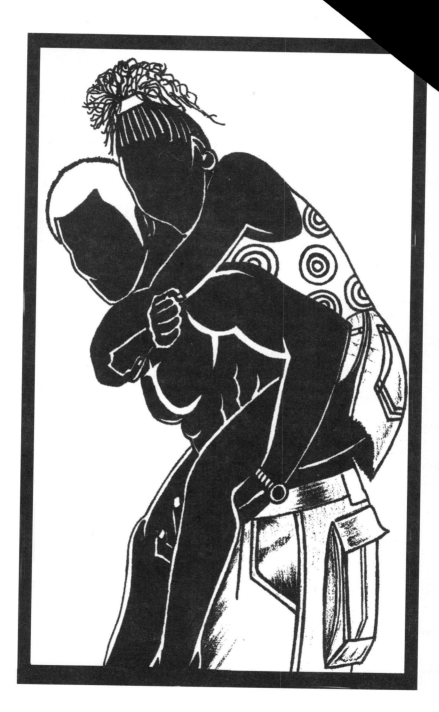

)WLEDGE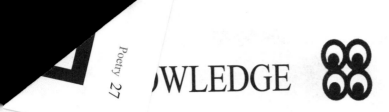

Knowledge   L
Kinti KOOL.
Coast to coast kinky coiffures KOOL.
Knowing MLK and knowing one's history KOOL.
K W A N Z A A Kujichagalugia Kuumba KOOL.

KINGS and QUEENS and POWER and THINGS.

Knowing about the Kundalini KOOL.
Keep Kingdoms keys.
Keen clever karma.
Kinship, kindred, kinfolk KOOL.

KINGS and QUEENS and POWER and THINGS.

KIDS, no one can kill, kidnap nor confiscate knowledge.
Kemet.
Kismet.
Keep your heads up and keep kicking colossal kilowatts kinetically.

Kudos!

Leaders Love Light

Leaders LOVE Light.
Live luminous lives.
LIFE FORCE, lifetimes, long lasting lineage.
Legendary like lions.
Loom, live large.

Leaders LIBERATE.
Lay laws and lock loud loose lips and lift language.
Legal license.
Limit lack, limit lies, limit laziness, loneliness and lawlessness.
Leverage self-knowingness, logon laser ladyluck.
LEADERS LEAD!

LEADERS LORD LOVE!
Like the lovely lotus blossoms.
Lessen lectures, lavish lore.
Loopin lofty lyrics, literature and libations to the legends.
Laugh.
Locate lifeguards to locate Lost cubs.
Look for longevity.
Look for loyalty.

LITTLE LEADERS LISTEN.
Learn lessons.
Love life.
Let live.

LEAVE LASTING LEGACY.

Mothers Mission

MOTHERS Mission MOVE Mountains.
MAAT ... MOTHERLAND'S MYSTICAL Matrix memory.
Metaphysical molecular melanin muscle.
Modern Moms meditate and create mantras.
MINDFULNESS MANIFESTS MIRACLES.
Mmmmmortality.
Moms make mistakes.
Missed mother's medicine, missed mother's milk.

MILLENNIUM Message for the masses.
MAKE MOTHERHOOD MAGNIFICENT!
Marry mature mate.
Marriage means matrimony ... must maintain.
Matriarchs merits morals, merits magnification.
Mmmmmotherlode.

Mothers, martyrs and mentors must manage money and maximize.
Master mind blind man's markets and monopolize.
Mothers must motivate members for a micro macro movement
non-materialistic mathematical mindset.
Mmmmm MAYBE A MILLION MOTHER MARCH IN MAY?

MOTHERS MANDATE, must monitor media's mediocrity maze.
Must make multinational mega corporations accountable.
Minority mix mostly manipulated and misrepresented.
Majors making megabytes and megabucks.
Momma's babies mimicking MTV & movies, marginalizing morality,
making immobilized mis-educated mopes and "at risk" maniacs.

MERCY, MERCY MERCY ME!

Dark Chocolate, Cinnamon, Nutmeg, Ginger, Mocha Mindful Moms.
Make more memorable MAD MUSIC.
More MIRACLES,
More mighty manna,
More MAGIC MOMENTS ... My Lady MOMMA Love.

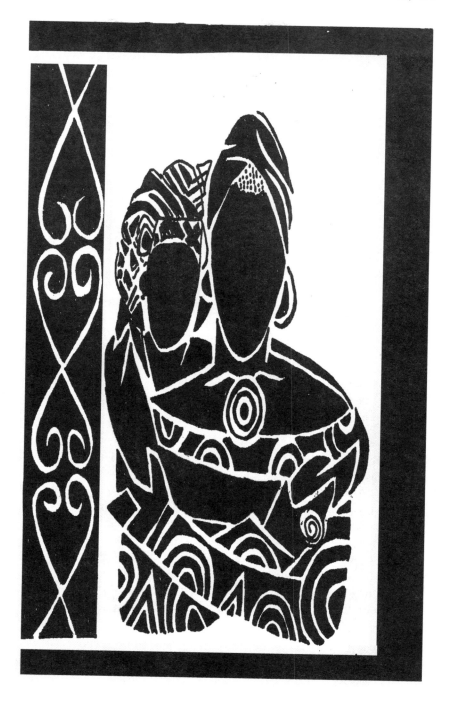

NOTICE

Never   Neglect   NEIGHBORHOODS.
NEUTRALIZE NEGATIVE ENERGY.
Natives negligent nowadays.
Need to know about environmental racism and toxic dumps
numbering our neighborhoods near our schools and homes.
Nuclear waste nilating Negroes and making naive folk nervous,
nauseous, nearsighted and leaving them numb and alone.
Nonstop noise and narcotics makes neurotic niggas hate and rage.
Nothing is sacred, they never knew their history and now all they
want is some new Nikes and to get paid.

Need nice nest ... nature's natural ... nurture neighborliness now.

NGUZO SABA ... network and get it together on the INTERNET.
And start communicating and organizing international corporations
and social political race relations.
Narrowing known slacken hackers entrances and access.
NEED NET PROTECTION AND GOOD VIRUS DETECTION.
Notice the direction.
Next level of denial of access for all conscious Africans.
Nixing nubians privacy, falsifying your information and nullifying your
reputation.

Need nice nest ... nature's natural ... nurture neighborliness now.

Nia NOW!
Need NAPPY NUBIAN NOBLE KNIGHTS now.
Nubian NOBILITY needs nurturing now!
NEIGHBORHOODS are the NUCLEUS.
Nubian Noble Knights not nomads, not niggas ... nonsense!
Noble Knights stop knockin and start innoculatin the neighborhood.
Noone wants to live in an unsafe unkempt uncared for space.
Now you name it!
NUBIAN NATION NECESSARY!

ONLINE OBJECTIVE

Overcome obsolete obstacles.

Over turn outdated old opinions.

Organize thoughts and outshine opponent.

Obliterate obnoxious obscenities, obsessions and oppressions.

Outsmart overpower and oust outlaws.

Object, oppose and ostrasize for the cause.

Operate only on obedient oneness.

Orbit outerspace and observe organic order.

Outcome optimistic.

Orisa's and ORIGINAL People's origins.

Ori Ori Ori!

Ode to the odyssey our obligation.

Own up open up ... Orunmila, Ogun, Obatalla, Oya, Olukun, Yemonja, Osun, Esu and Sango!

Only one Oludumare.

Our Divine Creator.

Omnipotent, Omniscient, Omnipresent.

PEER PRESSURE

Peer pressure ... POWER PLAY.
Plays people.
Past and present.
Promise, preface point.
Probably puzzled person and posse protesting planetary paranoid personality.
Poo don't believe it.
Peep this.

PEER PRESSURE'S PLAIN PUSHIN!
Peer pressure polarizes people's potential and plucks at self-esteem.
Peers pressure and persuade you to follow and not lead.
Papow ... price to pay.

PERFECT PLAN pardon the push.
Psychoanalyze, ponder position and pick profile.
Political, popular, principled, programmed, partyer, primitive, punkish, perpetrator, patriotic or plain prejudice?
Project positive presence to the playas and plant the seed.
Prepare to protect power place.

PATIENCE, PICTURE PRIDE.
Purposefully proceed personal path.
Persistence pays off ... pain passes ... persevere.
Practicing PRAYER promotes phat platinum promise, prosperity and praises from your peoples ... props!

Parents particularly proud of progeny's personhood.
P.S. PLANNING PREGNANCY precedes progress.
Plan to prioritize PARENTHOOD.
Proclaim Abstinence, Stay in School and Pursue Your Dreams.
PEACE.

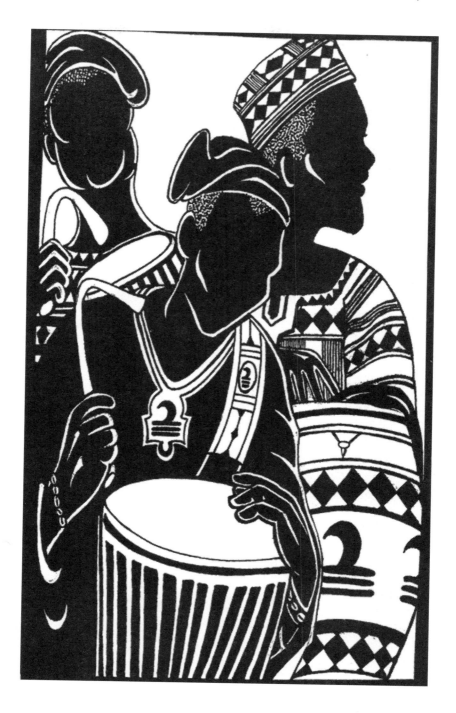

Quick Quotes

QUEST quickens quite quickly.

QUIT quarreling.

QUIT quibbling.

QUIT the chitty chatter.

QUIET!

QUERY the messenger.

QUIZ the teacher.

QUALIFY the history books.

QUEEN the Queens and King the Kings and quote the truth.

QUELL the crazy exploits in the melodies.

QUARANTINE the illegal substances in the community.

QUAKE the unconscious sistas and brothas.

QUANTIFY the government's hidden agendas.

QUASH the media's masked motivation.

QUESTION authority's quid pro quo qualifications.

QUESTION the system.

QUESTION your conscious.

Respect

RECEIVE REAL RESPECT.
Rape is wrong.
Remain responsible, rap it up relationships are important.
Resilience reigns.
Remember RECIPROCITY?
Respect reproduces respect.
REPRESENT!
Rap and Rhyme, Rasta Reggae rhythms righteously.
R&B and HIP HOP religiously, just respect your Brothers and Sisters and of course revere your Elders.

Renew reputation.
Rewrite the rules RA RA RA.
Reawaken Africentric Rituals.
REGENERATE RITES OF PASSAGE.
Raises responsible children to adulthood.
Recognizing gifts and talents.
Radiates radiance!

Rebounding RACISM remains.
Reality is real, rejection is real, robbing rightful race.
RECOGNIZE it and realize right reaction.
Renunciation, repudiation, rebellion, revolution, REPARATIONS, redemption, reclamation and finally recognition.
Resurrect rich ancestral reservoir RISE.

Remember READING renders RIGHTS.
Reveals ROYAL ROOTS and reidentifies resources.
Reading reestablishes redefines and reclaims reasoning.
Reflects right attitude.
READ, READ, READ.
Reading reigns rich rewards.
Revelation ... Renaissance Rebirth.

SISTERS ✿

Sisters, so SPIRITUAL ... statuesque.
Seek soulful self.
Self Love ... SPIRIT SOURCE.
Sit still, stand stately, speak sincerely.
Stop all the struggling and start studying.
Study SHEROES significant skills and sensibilities.
Study science, study systems seek solutions symbolize strength.
Set SAT Standards. Streeeeeeetch ... STAY IN SCHOOL!

Show SOLIDARITY and stop sparring.
Stop stressing, stop smoking, stop social stigmatizing.
Snuff out stereotyping, silence sexism.
Social survival.
Secure scholarships.
SPECIALIZE!
Seek Bachelors Masters Phd's.
Synergize.
Sisters should know that the true meaning of feminism is self respect
equality and empowerment.
SUPPORT SISTAS.

Shortys, so shapely ... sacrifice stimulation.
Surrendering too soon ... SEX too SOON.
Slowly sucks sisters self-esteem.
STOP! STOP!   STOP!
SISTAS so SACRED.
Superior substance!
Simple strategy.
SAVE THE SEX FOR SOMEONE SPECIAL.

So until then, smile, sing songs, share stuff, share stories, share secrets,
stay sweet, stay soft and stay strong.
Surprise and SAVOR SUCCESS.
Splendid!

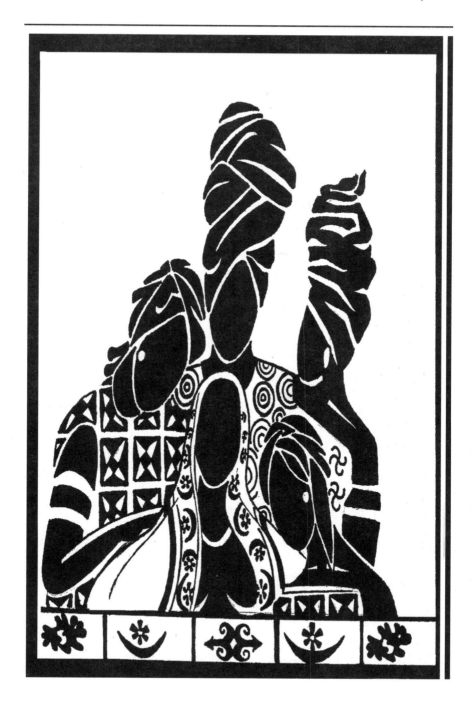

Today **I**

This time, teach the T R I B E tradition, trust, togetherness and tolerance through the TRUTH.
Trading the truth for a theory is tyranny.
TRANQUILITY tempers thankful transcendence to the top.

THOUGHTS TRANSLATE TO THINGS.
The body is the temple.
Treat it well.
Treasure it twenty-four-seven, three-hundred-sixty-five.

THIS TIME, TURN THE TV TO THE WALL.
Toxic tension trashes the mind, twisting intelligence thwarting total TRANSFORMATION.
Tick Tock Tick Tock Tick Tock Tick Tock.
Thugs time is of the essence.

THIS TIME TEENS THROW DOWN!
TAKE THE HIV TEST AND GET TESTED.
Total tenacity towards tasks!
Think, teach, trade, train, tutor.
Transfer TECHNICAL TALENTS to TECHNOLOGY'S TABLE to the twenty-first century.
Tomorrow's turf.
Tomorrow's throne and TRIUMPH!

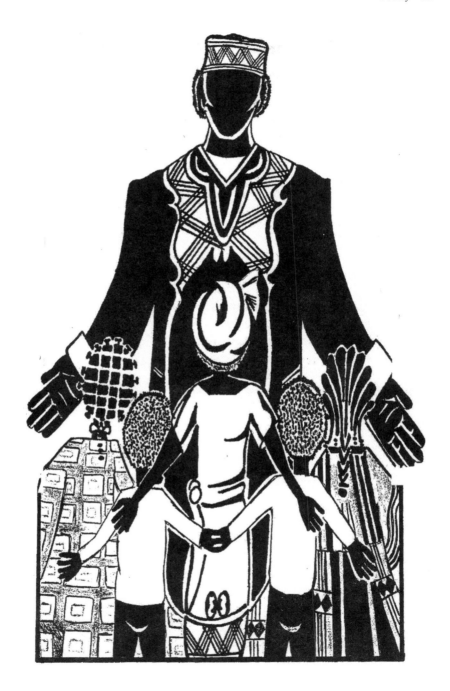

Urgent Undertaking

Unconscious and Unaware Unadvised, Unknown and
Uncounted Sisters and Brothers.

Unleash universal UNITY.
Umoga, ujima, ujamaa UNBROKEN.

Unity UNSPOKEN.

UPROOT, UNBLOCK, UNCHAIN ...
unfairness, underachievement, uneducation, uncertainty,
uncooperation, unexamined, unauthorized, unemployment,
unkindness, unfriendliness, underhandedness, unhappiness,
unfaithfulness, unforgiveness, unlawfulness, unreadiness,
unawakened, unexplored, unobservant, unmindfulness and
unfulfilled dreams and promises.

UNRAVEL and Unfold.

Utilize unified unconditional understanding.
Uplift united universe.

ULTIMATE UTOPIA.

Village Virus

Violence virus, visits VICTIMS, visits VILLAGE.
Virtual violent vibrations vandalizes all.
Violating all like a vicious non-discriminating VIRUS.
Visible vigil and veterans in vicinity volunteer and verbally vent voices.
Villains, vigilantes and visitors attend venting vendettas and their
vindicatory choices.
All vent vulnerability to guns, drugs and other socio-economic disease.
Vent anger and frustration at the veiled system, in a vernacular that
vaporizes the word please.
VOW TO FIND A CURE AND A RETURN TO PEACE.

Vanishing visionary valiant vanguard vigorously vote valid viewpoints
and a common VACCINE for the "Violence Virus".
Conjuring up ancient voodooistic solutions to bring healing, unity,
prosperity and trust.
Voting in the hood for VALUES, valor, volunteerism and vocations.
Voluminous variety of jobs and valedictorian training and educations.
Visible, validated vocal vertebrated representation at City Hall and D.C.
Versatile award winning schools and vast venture capital opportunities.
Viable ownership of their land and vested vertical businesses.
Vaulted ceiling homes with verandas and velvet covered furnishings
and very needed affordable healthcare and vital family vacationing.

Vaccine was applied and volatile villain's guns and drugs are verboten.
Everyone hugged and cried as the vexed vivid past was forgotten.
No more vices, violations, vulgar vocabulary, senseless fighting and
young people dying.
Only love and respect, good vibes and everybody collectively trying.
Vanguard, villains and vigilantes began to visualize and realize.
No need to take another valuable brother or sister's property or life.
Vintage Africentric Village is VICTORIOUS!
Vetoing violence is verily verily VIRTUOUS!
VIOLENCE VOIDS VISIONS.
Vengeance = Black on Black Crime = Everybody's Children.

WARRIORS

Warriors, when biological and economic warfare wrecks worlds, will
we wrestle with worldly weights, witnessing more weapons being
created for mass destruction?
And will we witness more unsanctioned wars being waged on the
poor and whine about widespread unchecked terrorism and corruption?

Will the well heeled wolves and warlords in Washington wave their
wallets waxing war games and politics just for sake of winning?
And will they continue to walk wrong ways harboring hate and greed
into the wilderness weakening?
And will their wavering wives and women who woo and wink, also
choose power and approve, without questioning, "What have we done?"
as the Motherland slowly closes her womb.

Will the wealthy waterboys want more markets, more wireless webs,
 more patients, profits and pills or will they become wandering working
white knights offering wellness and wall to wall HIV antiviral drugs
that can really heal?
Will their worst wicked fears finally wind its way back to their own
wild wild Western backyards?
Or will their wishy washy waywardness whip their wretched hearts?

WARRIORS what a whacky world ...who wants more hue man waste?
Who is willing to take a stand for justice and who is going to wait?
WARRIORS who's watching ... we do have a witness.
Wordup, whassup and what about the most high's divine wishes?
WALK WITHIN AND WORSHIP HIM.
And be mindful that the ancestors are always listenin.

Written ancient words washes the Motherland's wounds and worries.
Whispering healing wind warns sweet and warmly.
"Wear wings in unity brothers and sisters, weave wholeness and
welcome WISDOM."

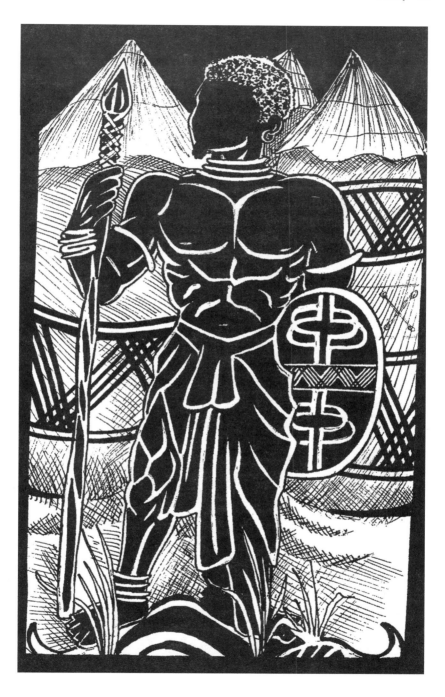

X

Xtolled

Xpansive

Xpert

Xclamatory

Xcellence and

Xtraordinary

Xpressions

Xceed

X's

Xperience.

Yesterday's

YOUR Yearnings yielded YIN YANG.

Youngbloods, you yanked it.

Yet your YOUTH yenned

YAHWEH'S yoke.

Yes

You're young.

Ya still got time.

Zany Zealots

Zany Zealots,

   Zooted Zooties,

      ZAPPED ZEST,

         ZIPPED ZOOM and

            Zig zagged to

               ZERO'S ZONE.

               ZOUNDS scary now what!

            (Remember Mindfulness)

         ZEAL leads Zygotes to

      ZENITH.

(Never give-up)

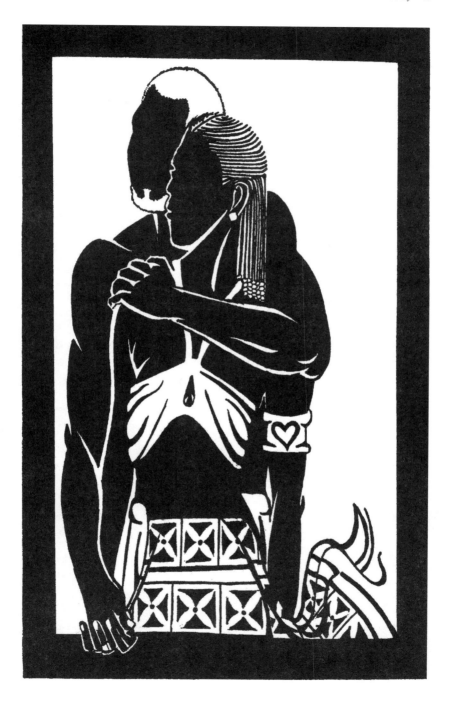

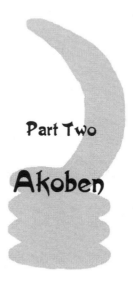

Part Two

Akoben

Akoben

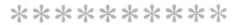

"Announcing AIDS Awareness ... AIDS Alert"

Akoben is an Adinkra word from the language of the Akan people of Western Africa. It symbolizes the sounding of the war horn and it means a "call to action." And this is exactly what we must do now, arm ourselves with "self knowledge" and prepare for battle because the AIDS epidemic is in full force. AIDS is short for acquired immno deficiency syndrome. AIDS is an aggressive disease that can kill you if contracted from someone who is infected. It is a deadly disease that is still incurable despite the discovery of new antiviral medications. Put bluntly, the AIDS epidemic is a monster on the loose and the battlefield is the <u>uninformed</u> African American community.

National statistics from the Centers for Disease Control and Prevention (CDC) reveal who is being attacked and notes the casualties. From 1981 to December 2002, according to the CDC approximately 886,575 Americans have been diagnosed with AIDS in this country and over half a million have already died. Currently there are 384,906 Americans living with AIDS and about 144,000 living with HIV (human immuno deficiency virus), the virus that causes AIDS. **In comparison with other ethnic groups, African Americans accounted for 162, 412 cases or 42% of the cumulative total number of people living with AIDS, Caucasians are 37%, Hispanics, are 20%, Asians are 1% and Native Americans are 1%. Also in 2002, the CDC reported 34,727 new HIV cases. African Americans were 50% of those cases (9734 males and 7134 females) and showed noticeable increase in infections among 13 to 24 year olds. These statistics are quite scary and should be of concern to everyone especially when one**

considers that African Americans are only 13% of the total U.S. Population.

The picture is even worse when we look at what is happening to our brothers and sisters in the Motherland. **Already, more than 29 million Africans are infected with HIV/AIDS and another 20 million have already died from AIDS related diseases.** The AIDS holocaust in Africa has orphaned over 14 million children and has turned once thriving villages into deserted ghost towns. In addition, the World Health Organization (WHO) is reporting a significant increase in the number of aids cases in India, China and Europe, estimating that there are approximately **42 million people infected with HIV/AIDS worldwide. Is this not a wake up call?** And what if any is the underlying message to this epidemic?

Scientists have been tracking AIDS, as we know it since 1981, but the exact origin of the disease is still being debated. Some say the HIV virus originated from green monkeys. Others say it was created in a test tube and or it could have been an experiment gone wrong. In the early days, everyone thought it was a disease prevalent only among gay white males. However, when it jumped the demographic fence into the heterosexual population, America was not prepared. Early on, men and women of all persuasions were in denial and condom use was inconsistent. And at the national level, there was a lack of adequate programs to educate the public on how to proactively protect themselves and prevent the disease from spreading.

African Americans were also unprepared, as they had already been placed on an uneven playing field where they were constantly under attack from the proliferation of drugs, poverty, violence, deceit and unemployment. And still lingering in many people's minds was the 1932 Tuskegee Syphilis Experiment, when the U.S. government secretly injected 399 African American men with the syphilis virus and never provided any of them with proper medical treatment. For more than forty years the true nature of their illness was hidden from these men and their families. Which caused many of them great pain and suffering and to distrust the government.

No one can uproot the tree which God has planted.
Yoruba proverb

HIV/AIDS Near Our Schools and Homes

Now HIV/AIDS is in our immediate environment, causing generational havoc by weakening our families and communities with massive loss of life and increasing Healthcare costs. **HIV/AIDS is more serious than anyone could imagine because it Is also a threat to our adolescent and senior citizen populations. African American women are also threatened and are now considered to have one of the highest infection rates in the country.** HIV/AIDS is continuing to spread unchecked in all age groups through "high-risk" sexual behavior and the following situations.

1. Sex with multiple partners.
2. Men who have sex with men.
3. Men who are having sex secretly on the "down low" with other men and women but who don't consider themselves gay or bisexual.
4. Intravenous drug use.
5. Infection at birth (from a parent).
6. Blood transfusions (although rarely).

Anyone can catch the disease if they are not practicing safe sex or are sharing needles with an infected person. AIDS does not discriminate. Race and sexual orientation do not matter. Anyone can become infected. HIV/AIDS is an equal opportunity disease.

HIV/AIDS is on the move in the African American community because many people are still denying its presence and impact within our culture and society. **By choosing to be silent and refusing to admit that we are in the midst of a crisis in our community we do ourselves and everyone around us an injustice.** We cannot begin to heal as a people until we first acknowledge that we have a problem. Silence and secrecy hurts everyone. For instance how many of us know someone who died from AIDS and kept their illness a secret because they were fearful of what their family or community might think? Or how about the story of the young boy who went to an all night party and later found out that the girl he had unprotected sex with was an intravenous drug user and had been recently diagnosed with the virus. Or maybe it was the one about the businesswoman who contracted HIV from her husband whom she later discovered was bisexual and during their marriage had been involved in a relationship with another man. Sad stories for sure, one can only imagine how angry and hurt the victims must have felt.

Many African Americans are uncomfortable simply talking about the disease. This is more true depending upon where you live, because many uniformed people are still very fearful. For them, it's as if having an open discussion about HIV or AIDS will lead to rejection and or being stigmatized. **Holding onto such petty fears is dangerous because if we do not arm ourselves with the facts and become mindful about changing our behaviors, habits, life-styles and our beliefs about HIV/AIDS then we are all doomed.** This is why we must break the silence and bring the HIV/AIDS epidemic front and center and begin discussing the dangerous consequences of high-risk sexual behavior and substance abuse with our children, spouses, families and friends and in our communities. Along with an open communication mindset, we also need to find a deeper understanding of ourselves and learn to be more tolerant and compassionate towards those sisters and brothers and their families who are infected and affected by the disease.

One of the reasons the virus is spreading so rapidly in our communities is because many African American teens are having "sex to soon" or having sex before they are mature enough to protect themselves and their partners. I feel this rush to experiment is caused by peer pressure, lack of values and the heavy influence of "casual sex" from the media. Who could deny that radio, TV, film and advertising is using more and more sex to make money and sell their products. The intrusions happen so often that we have all become numb to what we see, hear and feel. But it did not go unnoticed because many women have been voicing their complaints for years about the effects of sexually degrading messages in music and TV and its effect on our children and society in general.

When young people see stereotypical images of "hot bodies" looking sexy or appearing to have sex" it sends a distorted message to the naïve that everything is clear and therefore they have nothing to fear. This message is internalized and the end result is often reflected in young lives being disrupted and possibly damaged by sexually transmitted diseases, incest, unplanned pregnancies, abortion, rape or other violence. Sexually exploiting images and messages are everywhere: in the movies, on TV and in the lyrics of some of their favorite Hip Hop music. Most young people have not had a chance to develop the social and spiritual tools to understand their sexuality and their behavior especially when their hormones have been activated "too soon." They are growing up in a fast paced world where the values of family and committed relationships intimacy and responsibility has either never been learned or has been trivialized. Certainly, they are not even thinking about the possibility of becoming infected with HIV/AIDS.

Little and lasting is better than much and passing.
Moroccan proverb

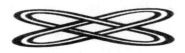

Youth At-Risk and "Boo and the Babies Too"

In 2001, a Youth Risk Behavior Surveillance (YRBS) for the United States was conducted by the CDC in 34 states from 199 schools to determine the prevalence of health risk factors for youth. There are over 3,000 high school students in grades 9-12 who participated in the survey: 13% were African American, 67% Caucasian and 10% were Hispanic. Here are the findings from this extensive report. (These figures have been rounded to the nearest percent)

African American	Caucasian	Hispanic	Total Nationwide

# of students who have ever had sexual intercourse during their lifetime

61%	43%	48%	46%

#of students to have their first sexual intercourse experience by age 13

16%	5%	8%	7%

#of students experiencing 4 or more sex partners during their lifetime

27%	12%	15%	14%

#of students who are currently sexually active

46%	31%	36%	33%

#of students reporting condom use at last sexual intercourse

67%	57%	54%	58%

#of students reported having been pregnant or impregnating someone

11%	3%	7%	5%

#of students to have used alcohol or drugs at last sexual intercourse

18%	28%	24%	26%

# of students reported being taught about HIV/AIDS in school

86%	92%	81%	89%

If these findings from the survey are accurate, we could say that the results represent the general climate for "at risk" behavior across the country for those student populations. The study also suggest that African American students experience sexual intercourse at a younger age and are more sexually active then their Caucasian and Hispanic counterparts. However, they also appear to be using condoms more and using less alcohol and drugs during sexual intercourse. Assuming this data is fairly accurate, it might partially explain why in 2001 black youth ages 13 to 19 accounted for 67% of the reported HIV cases even though they represent only 15% of the youth population.

The ruin of a nation begins in the home of its people.
Ashanti of West Africa proverb

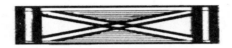

Wait ... "I want to Save the Sex for Someone Special"

Despite the CDC's alarming findings, **many African American youth "see the light" and are choosing to "wait" or delay their initiation in having sex. They know that having "sex too soon" can compromise their youth and maybe their future.** These enlightened teens look like the home girl or homeboy next door. Their profiles match their neighborhood and school yearbooks: they are hip hoppers, jocks, nerds, brainy, cool, street smart, gay, transgender, religious, spiritual, rich, poor and everything in between. What they share in common is a positive attitude and a high level of self-confidence in their choice of remaining a virgin and or practicing sexual abstinence. They are like other "enlightened" teens across the country who see waiting to have sex as a necessary goal once they are made aware of their options. In reality they are saying yes to their health and future and no to sex, drugs and uncertainty.

Still there are others who are sexually active and are demonstrating extremely high-risk behaviors. They are experimenting with drugs and participating in vaginal, oral and anal sex with no protection and often are jumping from one relationship or sex partner to the next.

Many think catching an HIV infection could never happen to them because they think they are somehow divinely protected. But they are very wrong. Anyone and everyone can become infected. My advice to them is simple: zip up your pants, get tested say prayer and consider abstinence. **The only alternative to abstinence is to use a latex condom correctly and practice safe sex each and every time. Just be aware that the percentage for getting HIV/AIDS decreases dramatically if one stays in a faithful relationship. But be "mindful" that abstinence is and always will be the best protection against HIV/AIDS or any other sexually transmitted disease.**

You can out distance that which is running after you but not what is running inside you.   Rawandan proverb

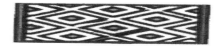

Drugs and HIV ... "Drugs Definitely Don't Do"

Drugs and substance abuse are a major problem in both urban and rural communities and drug abusers and offenders are getting younger and younger. Everywhere it's the same story. They get introduced to drugs through drinking alcohol and smoking cigarettes. Next they try smoking marijuana. From there it spirals into crack or cocaine or some other recreational drug, like ecstasy or methamphetamines. Some teenagers become drug addicts and are forced into prostitution and or criminal life on the streets. Others get caught up in selling or "slingin" drugs and sometimes become users themselves. According to the CDC, until 2001 intravenous drug use was the cause of 385 reported HIV infections for all youth between the ages of 13 to19. Also 1838 young girls and 183 young boys were infected with the virus from heterosexual contact. And another 1442 boys were infected from homosexual contact. Altogether 6588 young people (which includes all sub exposure categories) between the ages of 13 to 19 were infected with the HIV virus.

Certainly, illegal drugs breed negative energy within ourselves, our families and within our communites, resulting in a never ending cycle of moral degradation, poverty and crime. However, substance abuse has a direct relationship to HIV/AIDS and it is still in indirect primary cause of exposure to HIV across all ethnic groups. By sharing needles and trading sex for drugs one can easily contract HIV or Hepatitis C (another life threatening disease) from an infected person. Desperate people make desperate decisions that they later regret and using drugs will definitely put you in the danger zone. Also the short and long term effect of drug use can cause severe physical damage to the mind, body and spirit. Causing the eventual breakdown of the immune system making it vulnerable to diseases and opportunistic infections.

People who use, abuse and sell drugs have been the cause of most of the broken families, neglected children, divorces, bankruptcies, violent households and senseless deaths in our community. But who is to blame. On the world stage African Americans are not the major producers of illegal drugs. For the most part we don't grow the crops, we don't manufacture the chemicals and we don't control the drug cartels. The greatest role we play in the cycle of drug destruction that we can take ownership for is being distributors and consumers. We are not the real players, only the bystanders sitting back and slowly allowing ourselves and communities to be consumed. So, those of you who are part of the (Hip or the Hop) generation who think that partying, drugs, drinking and unsafe sex is OK, then do the math.   It's easy. Substance abuse and unprotected sex can equal disease or even death, because once again, there is no cure for HIV/AIDS. For more understanding of the HIV drug connection go back and read my poem letter "D" about drugs.

One doesn't throw a stick after the snake is gone.
Liberian proverb

Alcohol and Tobacco

<u>Alcohol is also a drug and underage drinking is a big problem for parents and teachers.</u> Teenagers drink alcohol because it is easy to obtain and they think there are no major risks. In the United States the legal drinking age (depending upon where you live) is 18 or 21 and underage drinkers put themselves and others at great risk. Driving under the influence of alcohol is one of the most serious dangers of alcohol abuse for teenagers because your life and others can be cut short in a matter of seconds. Fact: Every year an estimated 513,000 people are injured in alcohol related accidents. **Another reason alcohol is dangerous is because under the influence it can easily impair your judgment and put you "at-risk" to having unprotected sex or set you up to be sexually violated.**

Also, beware of those new trendy alcoholic beverages called "Alcopops" that are being marketed to young people. They come in a variety of flavors with fancy labels. The danger is hidden in the sweet taste, which disguises the taste of alcohol. Generally they contain less than 0.5% alcohol, but they are still illegal if you are underage. Also be mindful, at parties because someone could slip a drug in your drink just for kicks.

<u>Smoking cigarettes is very dangerous too because the tobacco contains over 4000 other chemicals.</u> The main chemical, nicotine is highly addictive and usually has an immediate effect on the brain. For many, smoking is considered pleasurable but when we consider that smoking is the cause of 400,000 deaths a year, smoking quickly takes on a deathly look and feel. Also African Americans are the primary targets for tobacco advertising and smoking is the major cause of cancer and heart disease. Young people start smoking because they think its cool and they continue to smoke because they become addicted. Once the high of nicotine wears off, they reach for another more potent cigarette … marijuana. **Studies have shown that young smokers are 100 times more likely to smoke marijuana and form addictions to more serious drugs like cocaine and heroin then non-smokers.** Its no big secret smoking is hazardous to your health.

Other Important Drug Information

Here is a list of some of the most common illegal drugs along with their description, street names and side effects.

Cocaine *aka* Blow, Snow or Nose Candy

Cocaine is an extremely addictive drug that is made from the leaves of the cocoa plant found in South America. In its street form it is a white powder that is snorted or dissolved and injected with a needle. It is a stimulant that makes people feel great and powerful until their high wears off and then deep depression begins. A cocaine addiction can also cause mood swings and can bring on aggressive violent behavior. Cocaine usage has caused many deaths as a result of cardiac arrest and seizures due to respiratory failure. Those who get hooked on snorting the drug over a prolonged period of time can damage the mucus membranes in their nose as well as the nasal septum. Some users get so strung out they unconsciously act in strange ways, such as repetively drawing doodles, picking at their skin and waking around mumbling to themselves. Craving the drug makes people do desperate things including loosing all sense of morals and respect for self and others, leaving themselves defenseless against "at risk" behavior and activities. **Do not be tricked by cocaine because in reality it is like a poisonous snake, and if one is to close, eventually it will bite you.**

Crack Cocaine *aka* Rock, The Chunk

Crack, derived from cocaine, is probably the most addictive and destructive drug of all time. In its processed form, it is pre-mixed with hydrochloride to form a free base, which forms into a solid rock substance and is then smoked with a pipe. The term "crack" refers to the crackling sound of the heated mixture when it is cooking. It also refers to the irreparable short and long term damage it can do to your mind. By smoking the drug the stimulants reach the brain faster to create an intense high. Over time crack use can lead to paranoia, depression, cardiac arrest, seizures and respiratory problems. Since the drug is inexpensive and very accessible many young people fall prey to its venomous addiction. "Crack Heads" or crack addicts become very abusive to themselves and others around them. Since its introduction to this country in the 1980's crack cocaine has left a deep wide path of destruction that has done an unfathomable amount of social, psychological and economic damage to African American families and communities.

Ecstasy *aka* XTC, E, Essence, Adam, Clarity, or The Love Drug

Ecstasy is one of the fastest growing and most dangerous illegal drugs for youth. MDMA (methylenedioxyN-methamphetamine) as it is often called, is a stimulant that is part amphetamine and hallucinogen (mescaline). It is a designer drug and it is made in a lab. When taken orally, the white pills or tablets can cause unusual amounts of high energy and visual distortions. Usually they are stamped with an icon or some other recognizable logo to appeal to teenagers. However, sometimes the tablets are fakes and contain other substances like amphetamines, codeine or PCP. Ecstasy also eliminates anxiety and suppresses the need to eat, drink and sleep. Over time it can cause severe health problems including, hyperactivity, blurred vision, fainting chills, disorientation, panic, anxiety, depression and paranoia. **Another lethal chilling factor is the possible damage to nerve tissue and the brain when it swells after taking the drug and drinking to much water.** Because it is inexpensive, some young people take them at all night "rave" parties to stay awake, not realizing their hyperactivity causes a loss of decision making skills leaving them wide open to "at risk " behavior. According to the Drug Enforcement Agency (DEA) over half of the Ecstasy sold in this country is trafficked in from Finland.

GHB *aka* Grievous Bodily Harm, Scoop and or Liquid Ecstasy

GHB (gamma hydrixybutyrate) was banned by the FDA in 1990. It is the main drug used in sexual assaults because it renders its victims helpless and unable to fight back. **Hence the name "date rape drug." It is a colorless odorless depressant that has a salty taste and it can easily mix with alcohol and carbonated drinks. It is especially dangerous when combined with meth-amphetamines and or alcohol.** Some of the side effects include dizziness, drowsiness, nausea, amnesia, visual hallucinations, respiratory, depression and coma. There have been many documented cases of GHB related deaths in this country. To toughen the federal laws against users of GHB and other controlled substances that aid in sexual assault, Congress enacted the Drug Induced Rape Prevention and Punishment Act in 1966. Make no mistake this "silent drug" is so undetectable you would never know if someone slipped it in our drink till it was to late.

Heroin *aka* 11-500, Tootsie Roll, Smack or Junk

Heroin is a very dangerous "narcotic" because it is extremely addictive. The color of heroin in its pure form is white or dark brown. It is produced from opium, which is created from Oriental poppy seedpods and then shipped into the country. Another form of heroin is made in Mexico and is called "black tar" because it is sticky like roofing tar and hard like coal. To get high, the heroin addict or "junkie" snorts the powder or dissolves it in water to inject into their bloodstream using a needle. **A heroin addiction puts a person at high risk to HIV and Hepatitis during needle sharing. Intravenous drug use is still one of the major ways that HIV is spreading despite the availability of street level needle exchange programs.** Sadly, in the last 60 years many talented African American jazz, blues and rock and roll musicians and artists have fallen prey to heroin and cocaine addictions that led to their decline or early death.

Inhalants *aka* Rush, Poppers or Climax

Inhalants are very dangerous because they are cheap, accessible and can cause suffocation or sudden death. Inhalants are made up of common household and workplace products, which includes aerosols, lighter fluid, nail polish remover, hair spray, insecticides and cleaning solvents. Most users sniff or huff inhalants to get an immediate rush. However, they fail to realize suffocation can occur if the oxygen in the lungs and nervous system is displaced and they stop breathing. It is no joke. Inhalants have been known to cause irreparable brain damage. **Chemicals are poisonous and they are not meant to be inhaled.** Certainly the warning labels are placed on the bottles and cans for a reason.

LSD Tablets *aka* Acid, Blotter or Windowpane

LSD (lysergic acid diethyl amide) is the most potent hallucinogen known to man. It is over 4000 times more powerful then mescaline. It was discovered by a scientist in Switzerland in 1938 and was thought at one time to treat schizophrenia. It is so potent it is measured in micro grams (a millionth of a gram). All it takes is a tiny bit to send an unsuspecting person on a bad trip for about 12 hours. Usually LSD is saturated on a piece of paper (a blotter), which is imprinted with colorful graphic designs. Or it can be found in tablets (microdots or in thin gelatin squares (called windowpanes). The effects of an LSD high during the hallucinatory state can cause severe impairment of depth, time and perception with objects, colors and sounds. **Making the user vulnerable to bad judgment and personal injuries. The after effects include acute anxiety, depression and "flashbacks."**

Marijuana *aka* Weed, Grass, Pot, Reefer ,Mary Jane or Chronic

Marijuana looks and possibly smells harmless, but it still is an illegal drug. In its street form it is rolled into "joints" or made into commercial cigars called blunts and then smoked. Marijuana comes from the shredded flower leaves of the hemp plant Cannabis Sativa. Some of it is grown in this country but much of it is imported. In some states marijuana has been legalized for medicinal purposes. However do not be fooled. Marijuana contains THC (delta-9-tetrahydricannabinol), which causes short-term memory impairment. **Because it alters the way the brain functions, one could put themselves "at risk" by the inability to think and act clearly.**

Methamphetamine *aka* Meth., Crystal, Ice, Glass

Methamphetamine is a very addictive and toxic form of amphetamine. It is created from artificial chemical substance and made into pills. It is snorted, smoked or injected. People who are chronic abusers are known as "speed freaks" and some of the side effects are psychosis, erratic violent behavior, picking at skin, auditory and visual hallucinations. Meth addictions over time can result in severe brain damage, liver damage, chronic depression, paranoia, lung disorders and other physical and mental disorders. Another problem with methamphetamine users is that their children are often neglected. Most illegal drugs are produced outside this country, but Meth is produced right here in the United States. Because it is cheap and easy to make, it is fast becoming the most dangerous drug in rural America. Methamphetamine is not only dangerous to individuals but it is also hazardous to the environment because the chemicals that lab operators dump in the ground are toxic. These chemicals pollute our rivers, streams, farmlands and sewage systems and is costly to cleanup.

PCP *aka* Angel Dust, Supergrass, Killer Weed, Rocket Fuel, Embalming Fluid, Dust, Fry, Illy, Wet

PCP also known as (phencyclidine) is another hallucinogen drug. It was originally created in the 1950's as an anesthetic but because the side effects caused confusion and delirium it was banned. Then it was remanufactured as anesthetic for veterinary use on animals and in 1978 it was banned again. Now all the PCP found on the market is made in illegal labs and most is considered impure because much of it is embalming fluid (the chemicals that they put in corpses). PCP is very dangerous. Pure PCP is white and is sold in tablets, capsules, powder and liquid form. It is laced in leafy material like marijuana or tobacco. Cigarettes and joints are often dipped in PCP and smoked. This is called "wetting it up" or "smoking wet". PCP mixed with Crack is called "Space Base." Although the names may sound cool and sexy, this is a drug that will only make you dumber and ugly. Here are the side effects. A moderate amount of this illegal drug can cause extreme disassociation with your surroundings, numbness of the extremities, slurred speech and a loss of coordination. Users also sometimes feel a heightened sense of strength, exaggerated movements, profuse sweating, high blood pressure which can produce feelings of anger and rage. Others have been known to experience amnesia, memory loss, hallucinations, blurred vision, vomiting, depression, mood disorders and a psychosis similar to schizophrenia. **Also for adolescents, PCP can interfere with the hormones related to normal growth and development as well as those hormones associated with learning processes.** PCP is a nasty drug that is a threat to so many vital bodily functions. Taking PCP will definitely place you in an immediate danger zone.

Yaba *aka* Crazy Medicine, Nazi Speed, Hitler's Drug

Yaba is a high-risk methamphetamine base drug from Thailand. It is also called Nazi speed, because a German scientist created it originally during World War II to increase the endurance of their soldiers. Yaba pills or tablets are very small in size, but they can pack a devastating punch and can cause sudden death. They are manufactured sometimes in grape, orange, and vanilla flavors to look and taste like candy. **Even small amounts of Yaba can affect the central nervous system, which can cause elevated blood pressure, body temperature, irregular heartbeats, hallucinations, stroke or even death.**

One should keep one's eyes on one's destination, not on where one stumbled.
Yoruba of Nigeria proverb

However far the stream flows, it never forgets its source.
Yoruba of Nigeria proverb

"A Special Message for the HIP"
(Parents/Mentors/Educators)

✳✳✳

If we are going to empower our children with the facts on sex and drugs, we need to start helping them where they are while being mindful of where we want them to be. Given the urgency of the HIV/AIDS epidemic, it is imperative that we teach them how to stand strong in the face of peer pressure. Peer pressure is something most young people have a tough time dealing with at school because everyone wants to fit it and to be liked. But at what cost? With drugs and casual sex so available and visible to the public, many teens feel pressured to go along with the crowd to be accepted. Hopefully they have been taught a good mix of social skills that will help them stand confidently to communicate their values and feelings so they can set boundaries to ward off any unwelcome elements.

Theoretically we parents, their first teachers, should have been preparing them all along to handle life's difficult situations. But the reality is, many adolescent/teenagers do not have caring adults in their lives providing love, support and guidance. On the flip side, some parents are so emotionally absent they do not know how to communicate effectively with their children. Many young parents may not have had the opportunity to develop good parenting skills and or may have never been taught themselves. This is one more reason why young people are asking for broader sex education (sometimes known as life skills) courses from their schools and community organizations. They want to learn more about their sexuality, real life negotiation skills and their options. And they want less of the old-fashioned sex education lectures from teachers and counselors who are too often detached and unable to relate to the needs of the youth.

Ebonize and Edify: Sex Education and Empowerment

According to results from the CDC's School Health Policies and Programs Study (SHPPS) conducted in 2000, there are several weak areas in America's sex education program. The following facts represent all school districts and grade levels across the country.

59% of the students are taught decision-making skills relating to sexual behavior

68% of the students are taught how to resist peer pressure to engage in sexual intercourse

69% of all schools in the US require HIV Prevention Education

93% of the schools teach students how HIV is transmitted

95% of all schools teach how STD's other than HIV are transmitted

86% of all schools teach about the signs and symptoms of STD's

85% of all schools teach about the risks associated with having multiple sex partners

72% of the schools teach abstinence as the best way to avoid pregnancy HIV or other STD's

65% of the schools teach condom use as an effective way to practice safe sex

34% of the schools teach how to use condoms

4% of the senior high school and 2% of middle junior high schools make condoms available.

Nationally, our school districts are in need of improving their sex education programs. **Sadly, some school districts have ab-**

stinence only curriculums because they are still undecided abut the "need" to teach young people about condoms and safe sex. There appears to be a fear of teaching their students too much. Even though, the 2001 Youth Risk Behavior Surveillance indicated that 46% of the students in grades 9-12 have had sexual intercourse and 33% were still sexually active. The statistics and resulting "at risk" behavior are telling us that students are having sex with or without "enough" sex education. Which leads to this question, "Are some of the schools still teaching in the dark ages or are our children just not listening?"

I believe that healthy sex education begins in the home and parents need to seek better ways to educate their children regarding the basics of sexuality and the need to set boundaries to protect themselves. Then it would be dependent on the schools to provide a health and sex education program that included qualified instructors to teach both abstinence and safe sex education. It is also my belief that sex education would be more meaningful for students, if it were taught from a spiritual context, while being mindful to steer clear (for the benefit of school policies) of religion. **Such a program would also consider the importance of culture specific values, self-awareness, and self-esteem and decision-making skills.**

Truly, what African American youth need are more Africentric Rites of Passage programs during and after adolescence. These intervention programs could be organized by gender and structured to coincide with school curriculums, or as an after school program through a church or some other community based organization. In one community, several concerned African American parents and mentors saw the need to help young boys 14-18 and took it upon themselves to create their own unique Rites of Passage. It was successful because the parents commitment to the boys in the program. And also because the program's foundation was based on traditional African rituals, wisdom and teachings. Over the years, they have transformed hundreds of young lives and helped several "at risk" youth find their purpose and their path and finish school.

Just think, if this information and cultural experiences were available to all our young people at the right age and in the right dose, there would be less high-risk sexual behavior and less confusion on contraception, masturbation, intercourse and yes HIV/AIDS. The greatest benefit would be more confident teenagers and young adults behaving responsibly, and making more intelligent choices regarding their sexuality and relationships. The consequences of not empowering our youth with "self knowledge" leaves them more "at-risk" to acquire sexually transmitted diseases, become impregnated, be victimized by rape or some other sexual violation.

Also keep in mind that peer pressure is one of the major reasons for academic underachievement. So if your child's academic performance does not meet your expectations, be aware their grades could be suffering due to their peer group influence. Again get to know their friends because the older a child becomes the less they will identify with their parents values. If academic achievement is not a priority with their friends, more than likely it won't be with your son or daughter either. Be mindful that all of our kids have the ability (innate genius potential) to achieve and deserve a good education. With a little more effort on their part, surrounded by positive living and learning environments, provided by their parents and teachers and mentors they will succeed.

A mother lying down sees further than a child in a tree.
Krio of Sierra Leonne proverb

The way you bring up a child is the way it grows up.
Swahilli proverb

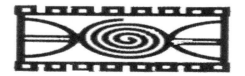

"A Special Message for the HOP"
(Adolescent / Teenagers)
✳✳✳

By now you are probably questioning just where this book is leading. What is the purpose of the poetry, pictures, proverbs, symbols and other HIV/AIDS data and information? And what is the point of the special messages to the parents and educators (Good observation because you are now moving into mindfulness.) All this information is designed to catch your attention and awaken your creative spirit because your health and well being are "at-risk." Already too many African American teens have sadly contracted HIV and it must stop. HIV infections will decrease if we stay mindful and prepared to make strategic choices about relationships, abstinence and safe sex. Hopefully after reading this book, you will see yourself as an informed "Mindful Messenger" and will pass this HIV/AIDS Awareness and Prevention information onto others and break the silence.

HIV/AIDS is in the House: What it is

HIV (human immuno deficiency) is a virus. HIV is transmitted person to person through the blood mainly four ways:

1. Sexually person-to-person through a man's semen, a woman's vaginal fluid or a woman's breast milk.
2. Tainted needles during intravenous drug use.
3. Infected at birth.
4. Blood transfusions (although rarely).

AIDS (acquired immuno deficiency syndrome) is the disease that is caused by the HIV virus. AIDS develops in the latter stages, after the immune system has been impaired and opportunistic infections begin to weaken the body.

The rain does not befriend anybody; it falls on anyone it meets outside.
Maasai of East Africa proverb

Silence is a form of speech.
Fulani of West Africa proverb

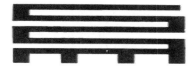

At Risk Sexual Activity: And HIV Infections

The kinds of sex that can transfer the virus from person to person include vaginal, anal and sometimes oral sex. Young people are more "at risk" of getting an HIV or STD infection, during sex when they forgot to protect themselves and their partner with a condom. And the risks are greatly increased when sex involves drugs and alcohol. However, many teenagers today think that if they are still a virgin and refraining from sexual intercourse, that participating in oral sex is technically not the same as having a real sexual experience. The fact is oral sex is sex too, and even though it is a lower risk, it is not entirely risk free. One can still contract HIV or Herpes from oral sex. Just keep in mind the more sex partners you have the greater your risk for becoming infected.

Young people also need to use caution when dating an older person. One would think an older person would be more responsible about their health and would be interested in looking out for your well being, but that is not always the case. In fact, they may be interested in you just for sex. Be mindful that an older person while more experienced has also had more sex partners and could have been exposed to the virus. If you are having sexual relations with someone who is much older than yourself, always practice safe sex and don't assume anything. And do not be afraid to ask them about their previous relationships. This advice pertains to both heterosexual and homosexual relationships with an older person.

Safe Activities and HIV

There are many activities one can indulge in with a person who has HIV/AIDS that are extremely safe. One cannot contract HIV from French kissing unless the other person has major bleeding in the mouth. Generally the saliva acts as a protective shield against the virus. Other completely safe social activities and situations involving direct contact with an HIV positive person include: holding hands, hugging, sharing food, colds, coughing, mosquito bites, toilet seats, showering or swimming together and donating blood. So don't start "bugging" if you know someone who has the virus. Remember to respect each other.

Safe Sex and Safer Sex and Safest Sex

Safe sex is making a choice to protect you and your partner from any possible STD infections and unplanned pregnancies. A person, practicing safe sex anticipates having sex and is prepared to responsibly use a latex condom correctly, before and after sex with all partners. Understanding that condoms are the only birth control option that also prevents the spread of disease. For extra protection, sexually active girls/women should definitely plan to use some form of birth control (examples: The Pill, IUD, Norplant, Depo Provera etc.) and spermicidal foam or gel (like KY jelly) should be kept nearby. Sexually active girls and boys should be mindful that the less they know about their partner the greater the risks of becoming infected with and STD. Also they should keep a fresh condom in their purse or wallet.

Safer sex could be defined as having sex with a loving partner in a long-term monogamous (one partner) relationship where shared feelings of love, trust, respect and commitment have been communicated. In this situation the couple has been tested and are using condoms and birth control until they know for certain neither one is infected. Or until they are ready to marry and rethink their relationship and future together.

Safest sex is and always will be abstinence. It is 100% guaranteed!

Abstinence and Celibacy Clarified

Abstinence as defined in Webster's Dictionary, is the forbearance from indulgence of an appetite and or abstention from drugs, such as alcohol or marijuana or cocaine to which one is dependant. It further defines abstinence as an act of "self restraint" and "self denial." So abstinence from sex or drugs is a form of self-denial. Taking it a step further, it could be called "self discipline" of the mind. If one does not indulge or participate in any kind of sexual activity including vaginal, oral and anal sex, he or she is being abstinent.

Celibacy on the other hand, also means abstention from sexual activity but it refers to unmarried persons abstaining from sex until they get married. Which explains whey the word abstinence is used to describe youth refraining from sex relations and celibacy to describe adults.

Personal and Private: What is Masturbation

Masturbation also known as "self pleasuring" is a form of sexual gratification some people do in private. It is the stimulation of one's own genitals or the genitals of someone else, for the purpose of obtaining self-gratification or achieving an orgasm. For all practical purposes it is considered normal and safe.

If you want sex while traveling, travel with your wife.
Minyanka of Mali proverb

OK I got the Message – HIV is a Serious Virus

HIV infections do happen and here are some of the symptoms:

* ★ Lack of Energy (chronic fatigue or weakness)

* ★ Severe or Sustained Weight Loss

* ★ Diarrhea

* ★ Swelling of the Lymph Glands

* ★ Frequent Fevers and Night Sweats

* ★ Persistent or Frequent Yeast Infection in the Mouth or Vagina

* ★ Persistent Skin Rashes or Flaky Skin

* ★ Short Term Memory Loss

* ★ Pelvic Inflammatory Disease in Women (that does not respond to treatment)

However, if you or someone you know has had any of these symptoms do not panic, they could be caused by other health related problems. But if you have participated in any un-protected high risk sexual activity and you are concerned for any rea-son, go to your doctor or local clinic or hospital and take an HIV test. (Most places offer free or low cost testing. Check the HIV/AIDS Resource Listings in Part 5. for a healthcare facility near you.)

HIV Positive and Antibodies

If one is HIV positive, the antibodies normally begin to appear in your blood a few weeks after being infected. Sometimes it may take three months or longer to show up. Keep in mind that the test for HIV is called an HIV antibody test because the anti bodies are the body's natural response or defense against infection. The presence of HIV antibodies in your blood does not indicate that you have AIDS. However if left untreated, the HIV will damage the immune systems allowing AIDS to develop. If your test results are negative, chances are good that you do not have an HIV infection, but if you are still not sure, call your doctor and take another test in six months. In the meantime, remember to consistently be absolutely abstinent or practice safe sex.

HIV Testing: Will It Hurt and Who Will Tell

Taking an HIV Test has never been more simple, convenient and confidential. In most states one does not need their parents permission. Nor can anyone but the individual being tested get the test results. All the information in the test results is kept confidential. You can get an HIV test from your doctor, at a clinic or via a mail in test kit that is available online for $30. (The results are FED Exed to you).

EIA (Enzyme Immunoassay) is the standard form of HIV testing on the market today. Results take about 1-2 weeks. This test is performed by drawing blood with a needle, which is usually painless. In some states it is still the main form of HIV test. The disadvantage to this kind of test is many people take the test and never return for their test results.

Ora Sure is another form of HIV test that offers accurate testing and is also painless. To determine if any HIV antibodies are present in the body, a swab is held inside the mouth between the gum and cheek for a few minutes. This test must be administered by trained HIV/AIDS test counselors in a clinical lab and the test results takes about 7-10 days. Again there is a delay but the test is quick.

Rapid HIV Testing is the newest form of HIV test to detect antibodies for the HIV-1 virus. It is important because they provide HIV results during the same visit and they are 99.6% accurate. There are two FDA approved tests that can be used in the United States.

1. Ora Quick Rapid HIV-1 Antibody Test screens for HIV antibodies and delivers results within about 20 minutes. It is administered by trained HIV/AIDS test counselors. Blood is drawn with a single prick to the finger and then it is collected in a vial and mixed with a developing solution. This method is quick, reliable and painless.

2. SUDS (Single Use Diagnostic System for HIV-1) another form of rapid test is used with a serum or blood plasma specimens. Test results are determined in about 30 minutes.

When a person takes a Rapid HIV Test and they test positive it is called a reactive (preliminary positive). Further testing is needed and always suggested to confirm the preliminary test results.

HIV counseling is available to anyone taking the test or making a request. During counseling, details are provided about the test as well as additional information on HIV transmission and prevention. Most counselors will counsel one on one, make recommendations and referrals and will also provide some literature. In depth counseling and guidance on HIV risk reduction is provided for those who test positive. Also the client is advised on where to obtain additional services and medical care.

The wise person who does not learn ceases to be wise.
East African proverb

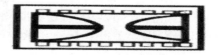

STD's ... HIV's Kissin Cousins

STD's (sexually transmitted diseases), sometimes referred to as STI's (sexually transmitted infections) are on the rise among African Americans and the target population is young people ages 13-24. According to the CDC, there are over 20 known STD's some of which show no symptoms. **The most common STD's are Chlamydia, Crabs, Genital Warts, Gonorrhea, Hepatitis A, B, and C, Scabies, Syphilis, Vaginitis and of course the most dangerous HIV.** Most STD's are treatable with medication, however if an STD is caused by a virus there is no cure. It will stay in your system and it can cause severe health problems including brain damage, cervical cancer, liver disease, sterility (the inability to have children) or even death.

The major STD's that are caused by a virus include: HIV, Hepatitis A, B and C, Herpes and Genital Warts. A virus that causes an STD's is passed through the blood, in semen and vaginal fluid during vaginal, oral and or anal sex. HIV and Hepatitis C can be spread by sharing infected needles during activities like drug injections, steroid use, tattooing and body piercing. In the case of Herpes, which causes sores on the mouth and genitals, the virus can easily be spread by just kissing and intimate touching.

Chlamydia, Syphilis, Gonorrhea, Vaginitis and Trichomonas are caused by bacterial infections. They can be spread through sexual contact and by sharing contaminated needles. All are treatable with antibiotics.

What is Hepatitis and Hep C

The most common types of Hepatitis are A, B and C. Hepatitis is an inflammation of the liver and is caused by a virus It can also be caused by overuse of medications, intravenous drug use, tattoos and body piercing, extensive alcohol abuse and exposure to industrial chemicals. All forms of Hepatitis can cause liver damage and some sufferers develop acute chronic infections.

Hepatitis C (HCV) is a viral disease and is on the rise in the African American community. HCV is a blood borne disease and can spread from one person to the next if left untreated. Most of the flu like symptoms are mild and almost undetectable. Symptoms may include mild abdominal discomfort, jaundice, vomiting and fatigue. Usually a person discovers they have contracted HCV when they take a blood test. Despite some of the new medical treatments almost 3.9 million people are infected with HCV in the United States. Until a vaccine is found Hepatitis C will be another major health concern for African Americans.

Be mindful that a person can be infected with a virus and can look healthy and feel great. Yet when they have unprotected sex, they can quickly pass a hidden disease onto the next person, just as easily as anyone else. The general symptoms of STD's include the following: sores, bumps, warts or blisters on the mouth, anus or genitals. Also unusual genital discharge, pain and burning when urinating, lower abdominal pain and general itching. If you think for a minute that you may have and STD infection please go see your doctor or visit your local clinic and have it checked out!

Before we get into the basics on condoms let's be clear on their purpose. Remember once again that abstinence is and always will be the best protection against HIV/AIDS and other STD's, so just because I am providing this information on condoms, do not think I am giving you permission to go out and start experimenting with sex, especially if you are practicing abstinence. Rather I hope the message you receive is that I am showing you how to protect yourself and others today and in the future. **So please for your own good BE SMART and continue to abstain from sex if you are already doing so, because it is the right decision, but if you are presently sexually active please remember to always use some method of birth control and wear a latex condom. There are no other choices.**

Condom Facts for HIP HOPPERS

Condoms were designed to make sex safer by protecting both partners form sexually transmitted diseases and unintended pregnancy. Their main purpose is to provide a barrier to block the exchange of body fluids. A condom should always be used during vaginal and anal intercourse. The condom that provides the best protection from HIV and other STD's is a LATEX CONDOM! (However if you are allergic to latex polyurethane is also effective.

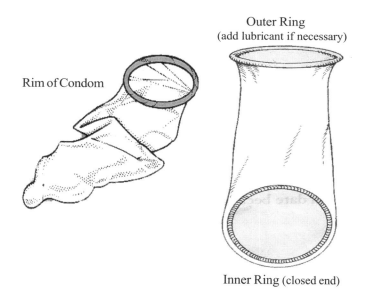

Outer Ring
(add lubricant if necessary)

Rim of Condom

Inner Ring (closed end)

Male and Female Condoms

* Condoms come in various sizes and shapes and are made of various materials, but latex is the best. Basically there are two types of condoms, the male and the female. The male condom covers the penis. The female condom fits inside the vagina and the inner ring covers the pubic bone.

The male condom should fit over the penis like a sheath. If it doesn't unroll smoothly then it is upside down. When putting on a male condom, start by holding the tip to squeeze out the air. Then proceed to roll the condom on during an erection with the rim on the outside. After sex, hold onto the rim of the condom and slowly withdraw the penis before loosing the erection. Before and after sex, be careful not to let any fluids touch the vagina.

The female condom fits similarly like a "diaphragm." Basically it fits inside the vagina and covers the vulva. For some, it may be easier to use for others it might be more cumbersome. Before and after sex, be careful not to let any fluids touch the vagina.

Condom Do's and Don'ts

Always store condoms away from light so they do not deteriorate and tear. And use caution when opening a new condom packet.

Never use condoms that have passed their expiration date.

Never use a condom twice.

If you are sexually active keep a supply of condoms.

Be smart do not take any risk. Use a condom every time.

A dental dam is a square sheet of latex that lesbians can use during oral sex to act as a barrier between the vagina or anus and the mouth to prevent the exchange of bodily fluids. They can be purchased in various colors, shapes and flavors.

When the music changes so should the dance.
Hausa of West Africa proverb

MOVING into Mindful Intervention and More

As a "Mindful Messenger" one has to remember to stay clear of peer pressure and the urge to participate in "at-risk" sexual behavior and dangerous drugs. If you do not want to experiment or be sexually active, when the urge arises, see it for what it is. And delete the thought no matter how good the person or situation looks. Be mindful to respect and protect yourself at all times and do not be afraid to walk away from unwelcome sexual behaviors. Instead take ownership for your thoughts, feelings and decisions and be your own person, with the understanding that you are moving into a new consciousness ... adulthood. And as you take charge of your life and make those moves, "represent" that you are responsible for your words, actions and their consequences. Continue to respect the rights of others and they will respect you back. Use common sense, speak your truth, find your purpose, set goals and visualize your future. (Remember the Ancestors are watching and anticipating your accountability!)

Young people must consistently step up and help move the human race forward. And it is especially important that you make choices in your life that will uplift "your" race. As you move into your own time of leadership and responsibility know that your accomplishments and achievements will not go unnoticed. Understand, that like your ancestors, you are part of this great creation and you are here for a greater purpose. Yes you and the Earth are and always will be sacred and it is almost your turn at the wheel. HIV/AIDS is preventable and so is drug addiction, violence, dropping out of school, unemployment and just about any other social economic condition plaguing our communities. Be mindful, the body is the temple. Treat it well and it will carry you gracefully to old age. You decide what thoughts and ideas you will entertain and allow to resonate in your mind. You are the master of your destiny. Choose to keep your mind, body and spirit healthy and disease free.

Also keep in mind that music is a good thing. It makes us feel good and it soothes our souls. But let's be honest, some of the lyrics in some of today's popular HIP HOP songs are terribly degrading and exploit sex and violence. Be aware of the "power of suggestion." **Over a period of time, sexually explicit music erodes our values and harms our collective psyche. Think about it for a moment and the affect music has on the minds of our little children.** They are listening too. Suggestion, take it upon yourselves to seek out conscious HIP HOP music or switch the station and balance your music tastes with some jazz and blues every now and them. (We created that music too and young folks need to claim and represent. If we don't someone else will.)

From here let me just say, you never know what will be your fate in life, but you and only you control your mind and attitude. But should you feel stressed or depressed or your thoughts are scattered, just take a deep breath and turn within. (You might even try meditation it works wonders.) The important thing is to take time to "know thyself" and stay mindful of all that you are learning about life. I was your age once and so were your parents and teachers. We did some crazy stuff too, but the world was different then and we did not have access to as much information as your generation. Nor did we have HIV/AIDS, crack cocaine and the Internet. I am glad I woke up before it was too late. But because of the bumps I tripped over during my teenage experience of "lack of self-esteem", "sex too soon" and "rushed relationships", I can advise young people on the value and importance of "waiting on sex" until one is truly ready. Guaranteed, the benefits and blessings of abundance you receive from denying yourself pleasure or an experience will far outweigh any hasty sexual escapades.

This is why I have included the Mindful Messages: My Choice to Abstain Agreement in Part 3 of this book. It is designed for teens and provides a text frame for making a commitment to abstain from sex and drugs. This agreement can be personalized and kept confidential or shared with others. Overall it helps prioritize your life before you decide to leap into a sexually active life-style. The beauty of it is that it clearly lists the positive reasons for being abstinent and it acknowledges love and respect for God, self and family over sex.

> Hasty marriages bring hasty divorces.
> Oromo of Ethiopia and Kenya proverb

Remain Responsible: Respect Relationships

For many adolescents/teenagers learning about their sexuality is especially difficult if they are also dealing with feelings of homosexuality (being sexually attracted to the same sex) and transgender (wanting to physically be the other sex) issues. If this describes your sexual feelings, do not alienate yourself from your family and friends. Talk to your doctor and or find a gay teen support group at church or at school so that you can share your thoughts and feelings. However, until you are ready for a relationship with someone special, take time to get to know yourself and get comfortable with your body. Learn to love and respect it, because it is the only one you have. Consider focusing on developing friendships. Real friends are there when you need them and friendships, when nurtured can last a long time. Dating should be fun and learning about your sexuality is a rite of passage to becoming an adult. But do not rush towards adulthood. Believe me it will meet you.

Being young is really a special time of life. Youngsters should not have major worries, (although unfortunately some do) like keeping a job, paying a mortgage/rent and paying bills. That kind of mental energy is for parents … they are the real adults. Young people should be using their time and energy to develop better social relationships and to explore their inner and outer worlds, beyond their familiar neighborhoods. Your mind should be filled with living life, positive inner thoughts and learning as much as you can about your African heritage, the world and other people. You should make an effort to hang out with your parents, mentors and enlightened elders in the community and absorb their advice and instruction. Good activities to give your time and attention to include: setting and achieving goals, learning new skills or a hobby, volunteering in the community, devoting time and energy to your family, friends, school academics and activities, college and future careers. And always remember to give thanks to the Divine Creator. Yes, this is the time to learn and have fun, but "mindful fun." Some call all this activity, "learning about your womanhood and or your manhood." Others call it just "mindfully" growing up.

When your quest quickens and you are ready for a serious relationship let your heart and higher mind guide you. Do not feel pressured by what your friends are doing and saying. Relax and be patient. Breathe! Meeting the right person takes time because establishing a good relationship with someone special whom you love and respect is a beautiful thing, (so is marriage). Soon you realize, you are worthy and worth the wait and so is your chosen mate.

Just take it slow and continue to develop and build your relationship with the qualities (love, trust, respect, communication, compatibility, character, spirituality, education, etc) that you most admire. Then one day you will realize that you are an adult and ready to commit totally to that special person and relationship. But again do not rush into having sex and keep the lines of communication open, use protection and everything will happen naturally and life will be good for both of you! Finally when you are ready, if your partner has been sexually active, encourage them to take an HIV test, before you two begin your relationship. It will give both of you peace of mind.

Where you will sit when you are old shows where you stood in youth.
Yoruba proverb

You must live within your own sacred truth.
Hausa proverb

I am HIV Positive and more Mindfulness

Should you take an HIV/AIDS test and discover that you are HIV positive or that you have been infected with some other STD, please do not panic and jump to conclusions. In the case of HIV, always make sure to take a second test to confirm your results.

The first thing that one usually feels is denial. "No this is not real," or "No this is not happening to me." Denial, doctors say is a natural response. But stay calm and catch your breath and ask for help. Just remember, there are professional caring healthcare providers available to counsel and advise you on your health and situation. **Just have faith and know that you are going to make it through this difficult time. It is far better for you to know what is going on with your health, so you are not in a position to unknowingly compromise someone else's.**

Before you share your information with family, friends or spouse think of how they might react when you tell them you are HIV positive. My suggestion is, the first person you confide in should be someone with whom you are close that is loving and non-judgmental. Remember you did not create the virus so do not be too hard on yourself. Be prepared for their reaction as deep feelings of shock, anger, betrayal, etc.quickly surface. Take time to gather your thoughts then take a deep breath and release any negative thoughts or feelings you may be holding about yourself or others. Finally reflect on your new situation and determine who may have infected you and whom you may have infected and plan to contact them as soon as possible so they can get tested. This is a very important part of the "mindful intervention" process. We have to step up and be completely honest with others and ourselves and do all we can to prevent more people from getting infected. Also stay positive and be mindful that HIV positive is not the end of the world. Just know that you are not alone and that HIV/AIDS is a disease that people can learn to live with.

Living Life with HIV/AIDS

****

There are many Africans and African Americans living with HIV/AIDS. You will meet a few of them on the next few pages. They are people just like you and me. They are no different than anyone else. They just happen to have a virus and or a disease for which there is not a cure. Some of their experiences are heartbreaking. Their ages backgrounds and in most cases the way they contracted HIV/AIDS are all different. One person was born with HIV, a few contracted the virus during unprotected sex and another became infected when she shared a contaminated needle. One young girl whose mother is HIV positive, shares her story about how it is growing up with a parent who is living with the disease.

While conducting interviews I found that some people were open to sharing their personal stories but were not ready to identify themselves to their friends and colleagues. Three people I spoke to revealed that they had not told their immediate families yet and were not ready to go public. Another was fearful of being discriminated on her job and also declined to talk. Others were more comfortable with their HIV/AIDS status and really wanted to help educate other people.

As their stories unfold, one begins to understand their illness and feel compassion for their condition as they and their families continue to live their lives with dignity and with a focus on staying healthy. Ever mindful that their experience and lessons learned are an inspiration to us all.

You must have love in your heart before you can have hope.
Yoruba proverb

***

Robert and Aimee (not their real names) were married in 1998 in Zimbabwe. He is in his late thirties and she in her twenties. They now live in the United States. They both have been diagnosed with the HIV virus. Robert contracted the virus when he became involved in a relationship outside of their marriage. This is Robert's second marriage. Prior to his marriage to Aimee, Robert drank socially with friends and colleagues. He dated frequently and did not always use protection. When he and Aimee met they both recognized that they were each other's soul mate and married about a year later, but Robert did not uphold his marriage vows. He learned in November 1999 that he had contracted HIV when he went to have some blood work done for a TB (tuberculosis) test.

He says that after he discovered he was HIV positive he told his wife the very next day. Even though he was still in shock himself, he says, "I was more concerned about how it would affect the people around me, especially my wife, and others who may have possibly been infected or affected with the virus." Aimee says that when she first heard the news she was upset but not angry. She also said that she became very sad and depressed because they were just starting their life together.

Aimee learned she was HIV positive three months after Robert's diagnosis. Her doctor discovered it when she went to the hospital to have a checkup. It was one of the saddest days of her life, she says. She became very depressed for the next two years. Some of her depression stemmed from being in a new country and living so faraway from family and friends. As of this writing, neither one has shared their medical diagnosis with any immediate family members. Not for fear of being shunned, but more out of not wanting to worry anyone back home. Aimee says, "For me the need is to be able to live my life. HIV has already taken too much of my life." Both feel comfortable at his point not sharing that part of themselves with others.

Both Robert and Aimee are well educated. Robert is in graduate school and Aimee is in the medical field. They came to America like many other immigrants looking for a better life and more opportunities. In Zimbabwe, the country in which they were both born, the situation is very tense. There is much political unrest and the economy is at its worst in decades. Ten years ago, Zimbabwe had a thriving economy and a stable government. There were no shortages of food, no escalated pricing and everyone generally seemed at peace. However, in the last few years under a new regime, the country has begun to loose the economic advantage it once enjoyed. Along with that they have been crippled by the HIV/AIDS epidemic that has already claimed millions of lives and seems intent on destroying the souls of all the people.

Zimbabweans are aware that HIV/AIDS is a national problem and it is a major threat to their country's public health. The most recent data indicates that 20 to 25% of the adults are infected with the virus and every week hundreds die from AIDS related diseases. This reality coupled with the lack of treatment and health care resources has brought with it a feeling of despair that lingers in the air like a thick fog. If a person becomes infected with the virus they are not outcast from the community like some countries in Africa. In Zimbabwe your family will help take care of you and offer what little support they can provide. "Still", says Robert, "Contracting HIV/AIDS is like a death sentence because there is very little hope. More often than not, a Zimbabwean will choose to neglect their health. If there is money it will be spent on food not medicine.

When asked why the virus continues to spread. One realizes as in other countries, HIV is on the rise because of the prevailing values and cultural practices. Mainly, HIV/AIDS is spreading in Zimbabwe through multiple sex partners and the practice of unsafe sex. Even though Zimbabweans do not believe in polygamy, there is a permissive attitude toward men having relationships outside the marriage. Promiscuity is a problem with African men just like it is with men in more modernized countries. In Zimbabwe a woman will not necessarily leave her husband if he is unfaithful. This lack of empowerment forces many women to stay in bad marriages even though they know it is possible that they could become infected too.

In Zimbabwe, young people are at a great risk to becoming infected too. Even though there is not a serious drug problem among youth (because there is no money and there is rampant unemployment and mounting orphanages) there is alcohol abuse and drinking problems. Like their brothers and sisters in the U.S., Hip Hop and Western media has a heavy influence upon them. Some kids wear saggy baggy clothes and dance to Hip Hop music. Although there seems to be a lot of information available to them, the messages are sometimes all wrong. Aimee says, "Abstinence should be common sense, but much of the abstinence education is loaded with judgment because it is promoted from a religious point of view. However, young people should want to abstain from sex and get tested."

Aimee believes that the solution to preventing HIV in her country rests with women and the youth and the availability of more healthcare. She says. "I hope America will do more to empower Zimbabwean women so that they have more control over their lives. Because for many women marriage is a means of survival not a relationship." She goes on to say that women and youth need more proper medical treatment at the clinics where they can be given condoms and supported on safe sex practices.

As they look back at their lives and think of their homeland and the family and friends they left behind, they are saddened because there is so much hopelessness. Robert believes that more studies should be done in Africa on people living with HIV/AIDS, but he thinks that a cure will not found in his lifetime. He and Aimee remain optimistic and hope that individuals in America will continue to send medical aid because having access to antiviral drugs is needed to save lives. This plea, they hope will be heard by many, because Zimbabwe, due to their independent political stand, will not be receiving any foreign aid from the United States government or other major sources to fight this epidemic. *(Interview December 2003)*

***

Hydeia Broadbent, the name Hydeia

means "Again". When I first heard her name the words "great idea" came to mind. This is what her adopted parent's; Patricia and Loren Broadbent were thinking also in 1984 when they decided to adopt a baby. Little did they know that the six weeks old bundle of joy was going to change the world with her ideas.

Today Hydeia Broadbent is almost 17 years old and has AIDS. She is also one of the most well known AIDS activists in the country. She has traveled throughout the world preaching and teaching a powerful message on HIV/AIDS education and prevention. Because she is young and was born with HIV, she can speak from her own experience about the many challenges young people living with HIV/AIDS face along with the difficulties young people have practicing abstinence and safe sex. Her advice to young audiences is "Make wise choices, stay AIDS and drug free."

Hydeia learned she had HIV by the age of four. She did not understand the full impact of those three letters but she knew how to pronounce them well. Had it not been for her new parent's love and diligence, she may not have gotten the care she needed. When the welfare department notified her parents that her biological mother, who was also an intravenous drug abuser, had given birth to a boy who had tested positive for HIV, the Broadbent's decided to get Hydeia checked. Prior to her being tested they noticed she cried constantly and never seemed to sleep or eat well. They also noticed that she was very susceptible to colds and other illnesses. The next time they met with her doctor her diagnosis was confirmed, she too had been infected with HIV at birth. They were also told she had only a dew years to live. This frightening news thrust them into immediate action and the search to find a specialist and the right medicine to save Hydeia's life.

Finally Patricia heard about a conference in Los Angeles on Pediatric AIDS. At the conference they learned about pending research at the National Institute of Health (NIH). In the beginning, she flew her daughter once a month from Las Vegas to Los Angeles. Once she was accepted into the NIH study, she had to fly her to Bethesda, Maryland every week. After that for the next five years, she and Hydeia made monthly trips so that her medical protocols could be administered. During the study Hydeia and her brother were given the experimental DDI drugs and were constantly monitored. Much of the time the medications were fed intravenously from a pump she wore in her backpack. Miraculously, Hydeia and her brother are alive today because of their adopted parent's quick response, the timeliness of the drug treatments and their own positive response to the medications.

Hydeia's speaking career began when she started accompanying her mom, Patricia to speaking engagements. Mrs. Broadbent became an advocate for AIDS awareness and involved herself in HIV/AIDS organizations. She learned in a harsh way there was a great misunderstanding about the disease, as she witnessed Hydeia being shunned and discriminated against by ignorant people. From then on she vowed to never keep her daughter's HIV status a secret. She says, "I couldn't hide the fact that I am black or a woman, so why hide my daughter's HIV."

In 1991 philanthropists Claire and William Milligan saw Patricia and Hydeia on 20/20. They envisioned a way to help and formed the Hydeia L. Broadbent Foundation to sponsor national AIDS awareness programs and offer education, prevention, community outreach and youth services. Standing by her mother's side Hydeia found her own voice and began speaking from her heart stating, "I don't want kids to have to go through what I've gone through. I want them to be able to tell people that they have AIDS and not have to worry about losing their friends, losing their moms or dads, or losing their jobs."

Now as the main spokesperson for the Foundation, Hydeia has reached thousands of adolescents and other young adults who want more information on HIV/AIDS education and prevention. They see her as a peer and role model and they listen to her message. Despite her battles through some tough times, including loosing some of her friends to the disease, Hydeia is strong and can withstand the pressure and hectic schedule of school and lecturing at colleges and churches. She is in good health and has not been really sick in several years. She maintains a daily medical regimen of a cocktail of 3TC, DDI and Crixivan four times a day. Even though her body size is petite she looks and feels great.

From time to time Hydeia experiences short-term memory loss, which is the result of brain damage from the disease. All of this along with being sick so much of the time delayed her formal education, forcing her to attend school for the first time in the seventh grade. Now she attends a high school and does most of her schoolwork from home via computer. As busy as Hydeia is she still finds time for her family, friends, parties and other school activities. She especially enjoys being big sister to her little sister, who also has AIDS and was adopted by Patricia. She also is dating and beginning to think of going to college. Even though her life is full she is committed to reaching and helping as many people as she can with a message on HIV/AIDS. She says, " If there were a cure for AIDS tomorrow, I would still live my life the way I am living it now."

Of her many accomplishments and achievements is the 1999 ESSENCE Award in which she was recognized for her AIDS activism. She was also honored by President Clinton, the American Foundation for AIDS Research, the Liz Taylor AIDS Foundation, and has appeared on Oprah, 20/20 and numerous other TV shows. Recently she traveled to Africa and met the First Lady of Ghana and other dignitaries. While there she also spoke to African youth.

Now that I have come to know her, the first words that come to mind when I hear the name "Hydeia" is light, courage and honor.

(If you would like to help Hydeia continue to spread the message on HIV/AIDS awareness and prevention please send a donation to the Hydeia L. Broadbent Foundation. Her website is www.hydeia.org.)
(Interview March 2002)

> Since the last interview, Hydeia Broadbent has received a Presidential Scholarship to attend Barber Scotia College in Concord, North Carolina. She is 19 and looking forward to going to college. Because her education is a priority, she is doing fewer speaking engagements. Her health is good, her optimism is great and she is excited about her future.

DaLaura Patton is 12 years old and

lives in Arkansas with her mother, grandmother and siblings. Her mother, Deborah Patton is 45 and is HIV positive. Deborah contracted the virus in 1999 while having unprotected sex. She told DaLaura and her 4 siblings about her illness when DaLaura was 10 years old. DaLaura's older sisters and brothers are between the ages of 17 and 28. DaLaura says that she worries about her mother being sick and prays for her to get well. Even though her mother generally stays in good health, there are days when she gets really sick.

DaLaura is happiest when spending time with the whole family, She loves it when her mom, dad, grandma and sisters and brothers all get together. But she also enjoys spending time with her friends and just being out of the house. She says that she does not worry what her friends think about her mother having HIV/AIDS, because most of them do not even know. When asked if her friends who know treat her any different because of her mother's health condition, she responded, "They would be more understanding if it was their mother who had the disease." She really doesn't like it when her friends start talking about her family. She says the thing she would like for them and everyone else to know about having a parent who is living with HIV/AIDS is, "No one should be afraid of HIV positive people."

To deal with her mother's illness, DaLaura prays for her mother to stay strong. Other than that, her life is as normal as any other 12 year old. She enjoys cheerleading and reading when she is not busy helping around the house. She likes helping others and one day hopes to become a nurse. She says she does not feel sad or feel that she has missed anything because one of her parents has HIV. Instead she feels fortunate to have such a good mother who loves her. But in the back of her minds she worries that her mother might die soon, because she knows there is no cure for her disease.

(Interview February 2002)

Since the last interview, Mrs. Patton's health has remained the same and she has become closer to her children. DaLaura is now in high school. She is getting more comfortable learning more about herself, making new friends and getting involved in school activities, including one of her favorite activities, cheerleading.

***

Carlton Wade is a 23-year-old young man who

was diagnosed on September 20, 1999 with HIV. He contracted HIV through a relationship with a man 10 years his senior. He grew up in Arkansas, completed high school in Colorado and now lives in California. Carlton knew at an early age that he was gay and found that being gay and living in a small own was not only boring but also dangerous.

Gays were singled out and constantly harassed. In high school he participated in the ROTC Drill Team and in other academic activities, but his home life was unstable and his personal problems seemed to overwhelm him. After his mother died, he decided to move to California to be with the rest of his family. In the process of becoming more comfortable with the gay life style he became infected. When he realized he was HIV positive he became angry, depressed and tried to commit suicide.

Eventually he checked into a hospital to get help and seek treatment. His sister was supportive and that meant a lot to him. When his spirits lifted, he reflected and took stock of his young life. His main concern became how to survive with HIV and go forward with dignity. At a retreat, he met others who were also gay and living with HIV. They shared their stories and directed him to a community organization that provided more support for HIV youth.

Now a Peer Treatment Advocate at a youth center in Oakland, Carlton sees first hand the problems HIV positive, gay African American youth have to face everyday. In particular, he says, "It is difficult for young gays to find decent housing and sometimes medical assistance." Carlton says, the two vocations he aspired to be were nursing and teaching. In a sense he is doing just that as he counsels young people on the importance of practicing safe sex and getting tested. He also teaches them how to take care of themselves. He says he is very motivated to help young people dealing with HIV and warns other young gay men to avoid sex with a person not wearing a latex condom. Carlton knows it is not that simple, because gay youth are especially vulnerable and could be easily misled by older homosexuals who take advantage of their naiveté and purposely fail to disclose their medical history. *(Interview September 2001)*

> Since the last interview, Carlton Wade now 25 has been diagnosed with AIDS. He has good and bad days but every day he must be mindful to take care of his health. After surrounding himself with positive people, Carlton's outlook on life improved. He also has found a best friend and has gotten closer to his family.

✳✳✳

Tim'm as he likes to be called, whose real name is Timothy T. West, is 29 and lives in California's Bay Area. He found out that he had AIDS a few days before his 27th birthday. He said he was not surprised by the diagnosis because his symptoms had started before he got tested. He admits that he was always attracted to men and had thoroughly dealt with the shame and secrecy that was imposed upon him by a "homophobic culture."

   In his search for himself and for love he says, "Ninety percent of the time I practiced safe sex, however, often caught up in the euphoria of being loved … I would forget to use a condom while having sex." He could have contracted the virus the very first time he forgot to practice safe sex, but then one never knows. Before Tim'm got tested, he was worried that he might never find true love and dreaded how his family might react to him being gay. He was also afraid of dying.

When he tested positive he said there was a sort of relief, for lack of a better word, because he was no longer dealing with the fear of the unknown. He knew exactly "what time it was." Nor did he have to stress taking the test every six months. Now he had to decide what he was going to do with the rest of his life. As new fears replaced old fears, he started taking medications and stayed busy so that he would not have to think about his disease. He got involved doing outreach projects and started setting personal goals. He also sought psychological help and began to find peace with God within himself. The inner analysis caused him to look back on his childhood and think of his family.

He was raised in the South in a large family that was headed by an evangelist. He is very close to his mother and siblings although his relationship with his father is still somewhat strained. He says, "There were lots of contradictions that I noticed between what people said in church and what they did in real life … and this was most apparent in my own home. We experienced domestic violence, poverty and worst of all to me, emotional abuse. But I decided that I would be loving, kind and good to others, often at the of my own wellness." Even though his family life was in turmoil, his Mother made it clear to him growing up that he was super talented and that being good at several things was a gift. This advice stayed with him and motivated him to complete his graduate degree in philosophy at Duke University.

Over the years his family has come to accept his gay life-style and are now supportive of him. Despite his illness, they have found new respect for him because he chose to share his relation-ships and disease openly with them. Since then Tim'm has gone back to school and completed a second Master's Degree at Stanford University. He decided to stop allowing the disease and a heart breaking relationship dominate his life. Even though there have been times when he has become very ill and the medicine was slow in helping him to recover, he maintains optimism about being alive for many years to come.

In refocusing his goals, Tim'm began writing a book and creating music for a Hip Hop group. His most rewarding activity is serving as director of an HIV/AIDS youth center in Oakland, called SMAAC (Sexual Minority Alliance of Alameda County). The center provides services that include safe sex counseling, access to food, shelter, medical treatment information and a safe environment for youth to "hang out" and socialize. At the youth center, Tim'm is on the front lines of the epidemic. Some of the youth he counsels are 15 years younger than he and they are dealing with similar personal problems and family issues. However, Tim'm learned about his disease as an adult whereas the youngsters at the center are just teenagers. Many of them are worried about their future and do not get a lot of family support. Some are living on the streets and many are jobless. Others are afraid and have emotional problems that require more in depth counseling than what the center offers.

Tim'm feels he is led spiritually to do what he is doing. He admits he would like to be more financially independent and often wonders if being so open about his sexuality and disease might affect his opportunities. Acknowledging that discrimination is real, he feels there is a blessing waiting for him. "Of that," he says, " I have strong conviction." People can say many things about Tim'm T. West living with AIDS. But one can also say that Tim'm, the writer, activist, scholar, emcee, educator and artist is truly a Renaissance man living his life.
(Interview January 2002)

Since the last interview, Tim'm T. West, now 32 has been quite busy. Recently he was appointed the Department Chair of a Public Arts Charter School. He also is enjoying the success of his new book, "Red Dirt Revival". He received an MA in Modern Thought and is working towards his Ph.D. at Stanford University. More of his "he/art" and music can be found at www.reddirt.biz.

✳✳✳

Ed Johnson started smoking marijuana at the

young age of 13. At the time it seemed like a big thrill, puffing on reefers and grabbing a taste of alcohol here and there, but who would have thought that this behavior would lead him to where he is today. Now approaching 40, Ed is HIV positive and recovering from a drug and alcohol addiction. Looking back at the last 25 years of his life, he realized the damage substance abuse has done to his mental and physical health. Not only has his health begun to deteriorate, but his dreams have been nearly destroyed too. Here is his story.

Ed is from the South. In his younger years, he was tall and handsome and always seemed to have himself together. He had problems like everyone else, but when he became intoxicated, the alcohol and drugs made him think he was untouchable. They also made him feel in control and he used them to escape from his responsibilities. Cocaine was his drug of choice and it also helped him attract the ladies.

Consuming cocaine boosted his ego and made him think he was the coolest stud in town. Soon he was partying regularly and sleeping with every pretty woman he could find. When he started smoking crack he knew he was already addicted to the drug. The more he consumed the more desperate he became. Once a drug dealer beat him up real bad and this brought him back to reality. After that violent attack, he realized he had serious problem.

Ed noticed that he was loosing a lot weight and his health was getting worse. He heard about the HIV virus, but because he was not gay, his pride and self-importance kept him from going to the doctor. Finally in 1992 he went to get tested. The two weeks that followed were the longest ever, but the diagnosis was confirmed, he was HIV positive. When he heard the news he was not surprised, because he knew there were a lot of naked bodies in his closet. He must have become infected from one of the women he slept with during a time when he was not wearing a rubber. He was just glad to know why he was always feeling weak and getting sick. When he told his family the news they were saddened, but because they were a close-knit family and believed in God, they agreed to help him. His family was not concerned about what the neighbors thought, because they knew he was sick. However, the drugs and alcohol were still raging in his body and soon he was back on the streets again. He could not resist the temptation and his family could not take his crazy behaviors anymore. At first he resented his family for quitting on him, but it turned out to be a blessing in disguise.

Eventually he checked into Decision Point, a rehab clinic in Fayetteville, Arkansas. There he had the time to detox and get sober. He realized he had three demons to face, alcohol, drugs and HIV, but with faith in God he would triumph. His sobriety birth date was January 4, 1993. On that date, Ed took his first step toward reclaiming his life. It was a humbling experience because inside he knew that God had not given up on him. Now he says that his main goal in life is to "Remain clean and sober and do whatever else God intends for him to do or need in life and be very thankful and grateful for it."

In 1955 Ed Married a loving woman named Mary. When they met she disclosed to him that she had the AIDS virus and had contracted the disease in a previous relationship. She was white and he was black but they knew HIV/AIDS didn't discriminate, so they never worried about what others thought. They were good for each other because they shared a similar medical history. She was comfortable and unashamed of her disease and she helped him to talk with other people and tell his story about HIV. They had a great relationship and really loved each other, but AIDS already had a claim on her life. After almost 4 years of marriage Mary was gone leaving Ed alone, but a stronger man.

He regrets not going back to college as he had originally planned to study law and play basketball. He also regrets that he wasted so much of his youth following the wrong paths in life. As he thinks about his own children and ponders their future, he knows their lives are going to be better because they are smarter and more informed. His beautiful 21 year old daughter knows about his disease and understands her father's situation. But his 12 year old son has not been told. Ed says that he is waiting for the right time to tell him. To support his children and pay for his expensive medical bills he works two jobs, one at a steel mill and another part-time with a youth group. Also, right now he is on medical leave and is recovering from a brain aneurysm. He knows he has to be proactive with his health to prevent more serious medical problems from occurring. Currently his viral load is under 400 (the virus is almost undetectable) and his T-Cell count is 986. Should his T-Cell count drop under 200, according to most medical diagnosis it would indicate that he has AIDS.

Ed has been living with HIV for over 10 years. He knows he has an incurable disease but his outlook on life is optimistic. He has met a lot of people who are either HIV positive or who have AIDS and he has seen some of them die. He especially feels for the young people who have HIV/AIDS, because he knows there is a lot of fear, guilt and shame coming from the black community, and he knows how difficult it can be to have to continue to work, socialize and lead a normal life without being shunned or stigmatized. He preaches safe sex and no sex (as he calls it) and tells young folks this, "Whenever you meet someone who has HIV or AIDS just remember, it's real simple, you are just like them and they are just like you. We are all children of God." *(Interview March 2002)*

> Since the last interview, Ed Johnson's health has remained stable. His viral load is 800 and the T-Cells are almost undetectable. He still works two jobs to make ends meet and he still has not told his son about his illness.

***

Chenita Smithwick is 45 and lives

in Baltimore, Maryland. She grew up in a middle class family. She is HIV positive and has been living with the virus for 16 years. Her troubles began in her early teens, which was also just about the time when she started hanging out in the streets and stealing clothes. She says at the time she thought she was cute and wanted to be a "Fly Girl." Her first sexual experience was at age 15. She dropped out of high school in the 11th grade, but by that time she was slowly graduating from snorting cocaine to smoking and eventually shooting drugs into her arms. She was completely turned around and had started turning tricks to support her drug habit.

During a time when she was sharing needles with other infected drug addicts she contracted HIV. In 1986 when she was first diagnosed, she was told she had the AIDS virus. At that time doctors did not know that HIV was the cause of AIDS and so they told her she had two years to live. This really frightened her because at the time she did not have access to the new AZT medication and she thought she was going to die. She continued on with her reckless lifestyle and kept her illness a secret for five years. She feared that if she told anyone she had AIDS she would be shunned and cast out of the community. When she went back to her doctors they discovered that she was HIV positive and did not have the AIDS virus. This gave her hope and helped her to change her focus and her outlook on life. In 1990, after years of drug abuse she finally found the inner strength to quit.

Now clean over ten years she knows who she is and has recommitted her life to God. She also knows that everyday she must take several pills to keep her immune system healthy. Today she is a peer group counselor for Sisters Together and Reaching (STAR) and travels the country doing workshops and lecturing. Her goal is to reach others by sharing her story and reminding them that they have the power to make the choices (good or bad) that affect their lives. Still HIV positive, she refuses to look at her life like it's a death sentence because in a sense HIV saved her life from a heroin addiction. She says, "HIV stands for Heaven In View and I now find peace and joy helping others and focusing on God with all my heart."

> Chenita Smithwick was interviewed over the
> telephone and her story was written, edited and
> completed on Jun 29, 2001. On July 11, 2001
> she made her transition. Cause of death … a stroke.
> She will be greatly missed by those that knew her
> and loved her.

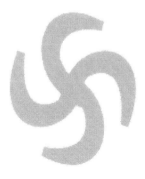

HIV/AIDS Call to Action

*****

This HIV/AIDS message is a "call to action" not just to young people in the African American community but to people of African descent everywhere. Although, some people are living longer more meaningful lives with new medications and stronger HIV/AIDS advocacy and policy, the disease still is the number one health crisis facing African people today. Being a woman of African descent, who is also a parent and a citizen of the United States I am very concerned about our collective response. We all need to be thinking about how we are going to address global HIV/AIDS issues that are threatening us and the world's most needy populations.

Many countries throughout the world are also battling with HIV/AIDS, but Africa has felt the depth and breadth of this disease. Countries like South Africa, Zimbabwe, Tanzania, Botswana, Zambia, Mozambique, Malawi, Congo, Kenya, Ethiopia, Nigeria and Ghana are being crippled socially, economically and politically from within by the sheer weight of the disease. In the southern regions of Africa, about 22 million people have died since the disease began in the 1980's accounting for 70 % of the worlds AIDS cases and 75% of its related deaths.

When I think about the longitudinal impact of the pandemic in 10 to 15 years, I am frightened because already for African people it is a holocaust. With no immediate cure in sight, how many more millions will die and how many more children will have to suffer the loss of their parents or grandparents? What countries will be the most "at risk" and why? Which population's seniors, men women teens, etc. will have the highest infection rates? Which ethnic groups in the United States will be the most threatened: African Americans, Hispanic, East Indian, Chinese, Native Americans and why? To what extent will HIV/AIDS undermine the economies of poor developing countries because of the mounting debt repayment loans owed to the World Bank and the International Monetary Fund? Which countries will get federal and international aid and why? Which alternative medicines and healthcare treatments will emerge? What long-term internal or external messages will the disease carry with it and how will that affect our social and behavioral patterns? Lastly, if someone should discover a cure for HIV/AIDS, would saboteurs undermine the vaccine to control world economies and or to make a profit or will they choose to save people's lives?

Who is to blame I cannot say? I can only hope that a vaccine for the virus is found soon and the number of HIV transmissions and the AIDS death rate trends start to decline. But until that happens, we must be proactive and recognize that practicing abstinence and supporting safe sex is the best choice towards intervention and prevention we can make for our health and our children's future. Inner transformation, compassion and healing must first begin within our selves. We all have a responsibility to prevent the continual spread of this genocidal disease and each and every one of us can make a difference. I feel obligated to give some of my time and energy advocating abstinence and safe sex for youth or anyone who will listen. But there are many ways as "Mindful Messengers" you can help too.

You must act as if it is impossible to fail.
Ashanti proverb

If we stand tall it is because we stand on the backs
of those who came before us.
Yoruba proverb

A united, conscious, organized and vigilant people can
never be defeated.
Unknown

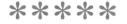 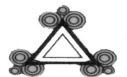 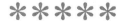

10 Ways for Mindful Messengers
to VOLUNTEER and HEAL the COMMUNITY

1. HIV/AIDS Awareness and Prevention education starts in the home first. It is up to all of us to be role models for our children and younger brothers and sisters. Get the discussion going and share this information with your family. Invest the time! Break the silence.

2. Our churches are the spiritual center and the main point of social contact for many people in the community. Get involved in organizing an HIV/AIDS Information Center at your church and help inform and educate the community. To get started contact the Balm of Gilead (an African American faith based advocacy agency) located in the resource listing in Part 5.

3. Organize an Africentric Rites of Passage Program for teenage boys and girls to build and strengthen character, life skills, cultural awareness, self-esteem and to prepare our youth for future leadership. Include a workshop on HIV/AIDS Awareness and Prevention.

4. Visit your local clinic and or hospital and spend some time caring for AIDS patients. Offer to read to them or seek other ways to comfort them. Let them know you are a Mindful Messenger and that you care.

5. Take a moment to remember those who lost their lives to AIDS and those who are still living with the disease and think of ways you can help. Also give thanks to all the dedicated healthcare workers who risk their lives caring for HIV/AIDS patients.

6. Find out what is and isn't being taught in your child's school health education program regarding abstinence and safe sex. Visit your child's school and get involved in their academic achievement. We need more African American teachers to teach our children, but we also need an African American presence from the parents, mentors and elders in the community within our schools.

7. Volunteer and participate in our local, state and national HIV/AIDS organizations so you can be informed and provide either your energy or other resources to maintain their presence and operations. Write your congressperson and demand that more money be spent on HIV/AIDS. Or get involved in an outreach program in your community and locate available resources and information on prevention, test facilities, counseling etc.

8. Reach out to our brothers and sisters in the Motherland and provide prayers, medicine and other resources. You can also help by connecting with an African Village or township through a national or international HIV/AIDS organization that is providing AIDS relief to Africa.

9. Make a commitment to remain abstinent or practice safe sex consistently and use a condom. Sign the Mindful Messages Agreements in Part 3. and begin your own Mindful Messages Ministry in your community. Talk to three people a week about HIV to help break the silence.

10. For peace of mind take the HIV test and encourage others to get tested too.

If you would like to get involved and volunteer your services or if you want to know more about HIV/AIDS, in Part Five I have listed a number of national organizations, professional agencies and websites that are located across the country. Certainly this list is not all-inclusive, but it can help to connect with the right services and resources in your area. Many communities have outreach programs providing HIV testing, peer counseling, prevention and treatment information. Some also provide financial assistance and shelter. Most are very caring and will also provide spiritual and emotional support, not only for those infected with HIV, but for their family members too.

The message is clear. **Married, single, gay, straight, young and old, we need everyone's commitment and participation to stop the spread of this deadly virus. Our children are all our future and we must all bear this burden in keeping them disease free and safe. There is much work to be done so let's get organized, digitized and mobilized before we are all socially and politically stigmatized.** Let's do our share in stopping the spread of HIV/AIDS and bring healing and unity to our community. Please all sisters and brothers, be mindful to speak to each other, hug each other, love each other and share this message. Ashe!

Education is your passport to the future, for tomorrow belongs to the people who prepare for it today.
El Hajj Malik El-Shabazz (Malcolm X)

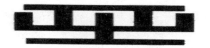

Real Facts about HIV/AIDS and African Americans

AIDS is the number one cause of death for African American men and women aged 25 to 44, ranking higher than heart disease, cancer and homicide.

One in 50 African American men are HIV positive. One in 160 African American women is HIV positive.

African American women account for 58% of the total reported female AIDS cases. African American males were 34% of the AIDS cases among men.

African American youth ages 13 to 24 comprise 15% of the overall population, but are 58% of the adolescent HIV cases and 44% of the AIDS cases. Black children are 59% of the reported pediatric AIDS cases.

African American senior citizens represent more than 57% of HIV cases among persons over age 55.

Intravenous drug use is fueling the epidemic in African American communites. It accounts for about 40% of the AIDS exposure in women and 33% among men. In addition, of the total 80,802 reported cases for female adult/adolescents, 39% were exposed to the virus through heterosexual contact.

Men having sex with men (MSM) among African American adult/adolescent men with AIDS represents 37% of the 218,349 total cases. Only 8% were exposed through heterosexual contact and 33% through intravenous injections.

AIDS is the leading cause of death in Africa. It is estimated that over 42 million people worldwide are suffering with HIV/AIDS. 70% or 28.5 million of those people are Africans. In the Southern regions of Africa,1 in 5 people under 30 are infected and over 12 million children are orphaned by the death of their mother, father or other family member.

Data provided by the U.S. Centers for Disease Control reported through June 2001

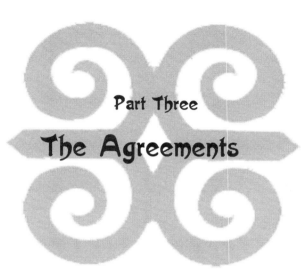

Part Three

The Agreements

Dear Parents and Adolescent / Teens:

The AIDS Message is a serious one and if you have not done so already, please take time to talk with your children about the dangers of unsafe sex and the HIV/AIDS epidemic. Our communities are in a state of emergency and the need to for immediate discussion cannot be over emphasized. If you are a parent who is talking to you adolescent / teen(s) about sex for the first time, be prepared. They might be able to tell you a thing or two about sex, You might be surprised to learn who your son or daughter really is inside and whether they are interested in dating the boys or the girls. By the way, did you know that by the time a child reaches 18 in this country, more then half of the females and three fourths of the males have had sexual intercourse? Or has anyone informed you that 7% of the students have had their first sexual intercourse experience by the age of 13? **In fact many teenagers are having sex and are holding onto their virginity, thinking that oral sex is not really a sexual experience and is therefore less risky?** And what about the recreational party drugs that are designed to look like candy that are fast becoming the new drug problem for teens and law enforcement agencies. Now do you see the need for making these discussions a priority?

Talking to your teenagers about relationships, drugs, sex and HIV/AIDS does not have to be complicated. Speaking openly and honestly signals to them that you care about their well being and safety. Be mindful that children are inquisitive and want to explore their sexuality, but most of the time are not aware of all the facts. Information on sex,drugs, HIV and other STD's can be obtained from your doctor, on the Internet or from one of the agencies listed in Part 5. However, if your child is already sexually active, and has had unprotected sex, do the right thing and get him or her tested as soon possible. It might be a good idea to have yourself tested as well. This is something we all should do during our annual medical checkup or as often as necessary. Don't worry, all HIV tests are quick, easy and confidential.

When the discussion on abstinence, safe sex and sexual behavior does come up with your children, parent's must send a clear message. Let them know that if they mix sex with drinking and recreational drugs, they will be at a greater risk to contract HIV or some other STD. Telling our children just day no is not enough. Give it to them straight but remind them they are spiritual beings and tell them how much you love and appreciate them. **Also, do a reality scan on their self-esteem and peer pressure points, because these are indicators of lack of self-confidence and wavering decision-making skills.** Assure them it is okay to be different. But remind them that they are responsible for their choices and the consequences of their actions, because HIV/AIDS does not discriminate but it is preventable

On the following pages you will see two written agreements, they are the "My Choice to Abstain from Sex Agreement" and the "My Choice to Abstain from Drugs Agreement." They are designed to help our young people increase self-awareness and stay focused. In this way, youth empower themselves by declaring that they are in control and committed to being sexually abstinent and or to staying drug free. (Such creative forms of expression are also a great way to strengthen family bonds.) In the back of the book there is a space to write notes during your discussions. Some teens may prefer to create their own agreements with their friends and school mates. This is OK too. The important thing is to get them to take that first step and make a commitment, the rest is up to them. However, if parents are providing plenty of love, (sometimes tough love), strong roots and sturdy wings, it may not be enough, but it will certainly increase their children's chance for a safe landing and a prosperous life.

Also in this section you will find simple breathing instructions that will lead you into a "Mindful Meditation" exercise. And you will learn of the many wholistic health benefits that can be gained from practicing meditation and mindfulness. Get ready to relax and connect with your creative inner spirit!

Mindful Messages

My Choice to Abstain from Sex Agreement

I_____,

make a vow and a promise to myself and my parent(s) or guardian, _____ to abstain from having sex until I am at least _____ years of age for the following reason:

1. I love and honor the Divine within me.
2. I love and respect my body and my self.
3. I love and respect my family.
4. I love and respect my people.
5. I am aware that sexually transmitted diseases i.e. HIV/AIDS, Hepatitis A, B, and C, Herpes, Syphilis, Gonorrhea, Chlamydia etc. could bring harm to future generations by damaging my health and could cause early death.
6. I am aware I could get pregnant or could impregnate someone before I am ready to be a parent.
7. I know there is absolutely nothing wrong with being a virgin and or being abstinent and I value my decision.
8. I am very aware sex is an adult responsibility. One that I am not ready for at this time in my life.
9. I know I am a spiritual being and therefore I will save myself and my body for that special person with whom I choose to share my love.

By signing this agreement and abstaining from sex, I am making an intelligent choice based on my Divine truth and I am embracing my faith in the future and myself.

_____ Date _____
Abstinent Teen

Mindful Messages

My Choice to Abstain from Drugs Agreement

I_____,

make a vow and a promise to myself and my parent(s) or guardian,
_____ to never do or abuse any
dangerous recreational drugs, including; tobacco, alcohol, marijuana,
cocaine, crack, heroin, methamphetamines, ecstasy, PCP, LSD,
GHB, mescaline, inhalants etc.

1. I love and honor the Divine within me.
2. I love and respect my body and myself.
3. I love and respect my family.
4. I love and respect my people.
5. I want to live my life to the fullest in the highest consciousness
   and be a part of a drug free healthy family, community and
   world.
6. I know dangerous drugs create negative energy and destroys
   lives and families.
7. I know drugs cause death and violence.
8. I know drugs kill dreams and I will not contribute to the
   destruction of our community and people.
9. I will not do drugs because I have great plans for my future
   and I want to_____ and
   _____ with my life. I also want be a
   _____.

By signing this agreement and staying drug free, I am making an
intelligent choice based on my Divine truth and I am embracing my
faith in the future and myself.

_____ Date _____
Drug Free Teen

Meditation is great for the mind, body and spirit!
Mindful meditation, when practiced daily has many health benefits.

Here are a few that will make you smile.

☺ eliminates stress
☺ eliminates depression
☺ increase your intuition
☺ increase your consciousness
☺ increase your comprehension
☺ increase your inner awareness

These benefits will manifest in your life for your greater good in the following ways:

♡ more focus for academics and sports (better performance)

♡ more self-esteem and confidence (likeable & good attitude)

♡ more compassion for others (less arguments and fighting)

♡ more creative energy (solve problems & make better grades)

♡ more healing energy (stay stress free, balanced and calm)

Mindfulness Meditation

The following is a simple breathing excercise that will lead you into a meditation that will help you to become more mindful (present and aware). Practice, practice, practice!

1. To begin, find a quiet place free from noise and distractions. Then sit up comfortable in a straight chair and relax with your feet on the floor, legs uncrossed and your hands resting at your side or on your thighs palms up.

2. For meditation to be effective it is very important to focus on your breathing. (Your breath is the key to life!)
Always breath in slowly and fully and to exhale slowly and fully.
As you breathe in, visualize the air as positive healing light energy filling you up from head to toe. And as you breath out, feel your breath as a letting go of unhealthy thoughts, negative messages and limiting ideas.

3. Start by taking conscious controlled breaths by breathing:
    in to the count of 4 then out to the count of 4 then
    in to the count of 8 then out to the count of 8 then
    in to the count of 12 then out to the count of 12 then
    (each time increasing the count by four until you are relaxed)

4. When you have completed the breathing exercises just stay relaxed, keep breathing and let your mind continue to observe its inner mindfulness. (If your mind starts to wander that's OK just focus on the air going in and out of your lungs and try not to think about any problems worries or other thoughts and feelings that may distract (your attention.)

5. Continue for 20 to 30 minutes or until you feel rejuvenated.
    (for best results do this meditation once a day)

Part Four
The ADINKRA Symbols

The Origins and Meaning of the Adinkra Symbols

Adinkra is the name of a traditional hand painted embroidered cloth from West Africa. It is highly valued and holds a special place in the lives of the Akan people. It is very important to the Akan culture and is a big part of the national Ghanaian artistic heritage. Here is some history on the hottest symbols on the planet.

According to some elders and scholars, adinkra cloth first originated with the Asante people in Ghana. A piece of cloth with a description fitting the adinkra design was cited in Kumase in 1817 by a British traveler. The cloth's actual roots, however can be traced further back to the Gyaman people from the Ivory Coast. The traditional story tells of a Gyaman king known as King Kofi Adinkra who attempted to copy the Asante king, Nana Osei Bonsu-Panyin's sacred Golden Stool. The stool represented the soul of the Asante Nation. The violation was considered an attack which angered the Asante King and led to the Asante-Gyaman War of 1818. During the war the Gyaman were defeated and King Kofi Adinkra was captured. The cloth he was wearing caught the attention of the Asante King. He liked the way King Kofi Adinkra craftsmen decorated their cloth and had his own craftsmen learn their cloth making techniques. The art form took the name after the King Adinkra and became known as adinkra cloth. The ancestors from these two groups along with several other ethnic groups that settled in Ghana and Ivory Coast became known as the Akan people.

The Adinkra symbols are geometric in form and represent a bold visual expression of the history, philosophy, religious beliefs, ethics, social standards, political systems and aesthetic concepts of the Akan people. They are part of their oral tradition and are based on historical events, proverbs, parables, axioms, hairstyles, animal traits, human behavior, inanimate and man-made objects. There are over a hundred core symbols and they are grouped into five categories which include: Animal Images, Human Body, Non-Figurative Shapes, Celestial Bodies and Plant Life. Their meanings are complex and multi-layered and convey messages honoring the ancestors and linking the past to the present.

Originally the adinkra cloth was designed and worn exclusively by royalty and other spiritual leaders for the purpose of sacred rituals and special ceremonies. When used in funerals and times of mourning, it renews the bond between the living and their ancestors and symbolizes the spiritual connection between life and the "after life". Today people wear both handmade and factory made adinkra. It is worn by everyone to many types of social activities, including initiation rites, weddings, naming ceremonies, church and festivals. Their bold design motifs are aesthetically pleasing and are excellent for making a personal statement on clothing accessories, tatoos, interior decorations, product packaging and business logos.

To make traditional Adinkra cloth requires several steps. The process begins with a special dye called *Adinkra aduro* that is made from the bark of the *bade* tree. Then pieces of fabric which are usually made of cotton are sewn together by brightly colored ribbons. The cloth is then stretched and held into place by wooden pegs. Then it is sectioned into quadrants by drawing two or more parallel lines. The stamps are made from dry gourds or a calabash with bamboo sticks attached for handles. These are dipped in the ink and stamped onto the cloth one at a time into various patterns. The cloth is placed in the sun to dry and then taken to the market to be sold. This type of Adinkra cloth is not meant to be washed.

The implied meaning of the word Adinkra is "There is a message from God for every soul leaving the earth." It also means "good-bye".

Take time to study the Adinkra symbols, you may find some interesting similarities to other symbols. One thing is for certain, they connect us to the Motherland and our ancestors and they provide a reservoir of cultural and spiritual knowledge.

Health ALERT: Body Art, Tattoos and Body Piercing

Did you know that the idea of adorning the body originated with people of African descent. Yes, body art as it is now called dates back 2160 BC to the ancient Egyptian civilization. In Egypt the women would tattoo symbols on their bellies to honor the fertility deities for abundance in the afterlife. The men also marked their bodies with tattoos. In other parts of Africa the Maasai, Dogon, Hausa, Fulani, Bantu and other tribes would pierce and stretch their nose, ears and lips and scar their bodies as part of initiation rituals to show status and social development and to distinguish themselves from other tribes. They understood and appreciated the symbolic purpose of the markings. For these people, adorning the body was an expression of self love and it enhanced the natural beauty of their skin, hair and facial features. Other civilizations that are also known for practicing body art include the Mayans, the Greeks and the Romans.

Following in the footsteps of the ancestors, the Hip Hop culture has caught onto the idea of adorning themselves with body art to send a cultural message of self expression. It is also referred to as body alteration or body decoration. Nothing wrong with expressing yourself, but if you are going to get a tattoo, get an Adinkra tattoo. (smile) For the most part, tattoos (except henna) and body piercing is painful, permanent and expensive. So, think before you get inked and know the health risks involved. **Because some young people have unknowingly contracted HIV and Hepatitis B and C from getting tattooed and other body piercings from contaminated needles.** So before getting a tattoo or any other form of body piercing be mindful to check that the shop is clean and reputable and uses sterilized clean needles.

The Adinkra Symbols

ANIMAL IMAGES

1. SANKOFA
(Go back to fetch it)
Symbolism: Revival, Revitalization; also Learning from the past to build for the future.

2. SANKOFA
A version of (No. 1)
Symbolism: The curved end represents reaching back to retrieve and revive the honorable and useful aspects of one's past, roots, heritage and ancestry.

3. SANKOFA
A version of (No. 2)
Symbolism: Respect for heritage history and wisdom of the elders, and a search for the positive aspects of the forgotten, ignored and concealed past.

4 DWENINI MMEN
(Ram's Horn)
Symbolism: Inner Strength, Determination, Humility and Strength of Mind, Body and Soul.

5. DWENINI MMEN
A version of (No.4)
The symbol also represents use of Power tempered with Patience, Humility, Tolerance, Wisdom and Discipline.

ANIMAL IMAGES

6. AKOKONAN
(A Hen's Foot)
Symbolism: Parental Protection and Discipline tempered with Love.

7. OWO FRO ADOBE
(Snake climbs a raffia palm)
Symbolism: Ingenuity and also the ability to overcome all odds.

8. FUNTUMMREKU-DENKYEMMREKU
(Double-Headed Crocodile)
Symbolism: Unity in Diversity and Ingenuity and Shared Destiny.

9. FUNTUMMREKU
A version of (No. 8)
Symbolism: The union of two contrary principles. The Man-Woman and the Woman-Man attributes of the Divine Creator and Creation itself.

10. FUNTUMMREKU
This is a joined version of (No 9)(Predates Swastika)
Symbolism: Duality of the essence of Life and also the Female-Male Principles of Life.

ANIMAL
IMAGES

11. ODENKYEM
(Crocodile)
Symbolism: Propriety
and Prudence.

**12. A version of
ODENKYEM**
(Crocodile)
Symbolism: Propriety
and Prudence.

13. ANANSE NTONTAN
(The Spiders Web)
Symbolism: Wisdom,
Ingenuity, Creativity,
Craftiness, Complexity
and Interdependency
of all Creation.

14. FAFANTO
(Butterfly)
Symbolism: Gentleness,
Honesty and Prudence.

15. ESONO NANTAM
(The Feet of the Elephant)
Symbolism: Leadership,
Strength, Power and
Authority.

ANIMAL
IMAGES

16. BI NKA BI
(Bite not one another)
Symbolism: Warning
against backbiting also
a need for Harmony,
Peace, Unity,
Forgiveness and
Fairplay.

HUMAN
BODY

17. AKOMA
(The Heart)
Symbolism: Goodwill,
Patience, Faithfulness,
Devotion and Endearing
Attributes.

**18. ODO NYERA NE
FIE KWAN**

(Love does not get lost
on its way home)
Symbolism: Love and
Devotion, Faithfulness,
and Endearing Qualities,
Fondness and Trust.

19. AKOMA NTOASO
(Joined or united hearts)
Symbolism: Unity,
Harmony, Devotion
Mutual Commitment,
Devotion and Family
Links.

20. AHOOFE NTUA KA
(Beauty pays no debt)
Symbolism: Need for
complementing beauty
with good character.

HUMAN
BODY

21. MPUA NNUM
(Ceremonial five-tuffs hair cut of royal functionaries)
Symbolism: Loyalty, Commitment, Dedication, Royal Spiritual Office Adroitness.

22. MPUA NNUM
A version of (No. 21)
Special hair cuts identify the rank of functionaries whose loyalty and vigilance are crucial to the security of the royal household and to the law and order in the society.

23. MPUA NKRON
(Ceremonial haircut represents the nine members of the Council of Elders who help the King and Queen to rule)
Symbolism: Democratic Rule and Collective Participation.

24. NKOTIMSEFO MPUA
(The Ceremonial hair cut of royal court attendants)
Symbolism: Service, Loyalty, Commitment, Dedication and Self Sacrifice.

25. NKOTIMSEFO MPUA
A version of (No. 24)
(The symbol predates the Nazi Swastika.)
Symbolism:The union of contrary principles, Dual Principles in all Creation Feminine and Masculine.

HUMAN
BODY

26. KWATAKYE ATIKO or GYAWU ATIKO
(A special hairstyle worn by the Kwatakye, war heroes)
Symbolism: Bravery, Fearlessness, Valor, Devotion and Recognition of Heroism.

27. ANI BERE A ENSO GYA
(Red eyes can't spark flames)
Symbolism: Patience, Self-Control, Self Discipline, Acceptance of Realism and Tolerance.

28. OHENE ANIWA
(The King's Eyes)
Symbolism: Vigilance, Security, All Knowing, All Powerful, Visionary and Introspection.

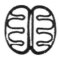

29. ESE NE TEKREMA
(Teeth and Tongue)
Symbolism:
Interdependence, Mutual survivability, Collective Work and Responsibility.

30. ABODE SANTEN
(This Great Panorama of Creation)
Symbolism: All seeing eyes represents the Divine Creator and the Divinity of Creation itself.

HUMAN
BODY

31. KOKROBOTIE
(Thumb)
Symbolism: Recognition
of Authority, Cooperation
and Teamwork.

**32. TI KRO NKO
AGYINA**
(One head does not
constitute a council)
Symbolism: Cooperation,
Participation and
Democracy.

MAN-MADE
OBJECTS

33. NSAA
(A motif in Mali hand
woven blanket)
Symbolism: Authenticity,
Genuineness and
Excellence.

34. MPATAPO
(ReconciliationKnot)
Symbolism:
Reconciliation,
Pacification, Peace
and Harmony.

35. NYANSA POW
(Wisdom Knot)
Symbolism: Wisdom,
Ingenuity, Intelligence
and Patience.

MAN-MADE
OBJECTS

36. DONO
(The Armpit Talking
Dum)
Symbolism: Praise
Appellation, Goodwill,
Appreciation, Wisdom,
Poetic Eloquence

**37. DONNO
NTOASO**
(Double or joined
Armpit Talking Drum)
Symbolism: Praise,
Appellation, Goodwill
Appreciation and
Poetic Eloquence.

38. MMRA KRADO
(The lock or seal of law)
Symbolism: Authority,
Legality, Legitimacy,
Law and Order and
Power of the Court.

39. MMRA KRADO
A version of (No. 38)

40. SEPO
(A Excutioner's Knife
or a Dagger)
Symbolism: Justice,
Punishment and Office
of Justice. Warning
against misdeeds.

MAN-MADE
OBJECTS

41. EPA
(Handcuffs)
Symbolism: State Power,
Law & Order, Reminder
of the ills of Slavery and
Oppression by the
Powerful.

MAN-MADE
OBJECTS

46. MFRAMMA DAN
(Wind Resistant House)
Symbolism: Fortitude,
Security, Family Unity
and Spiritual Protection.

42. PAGYA
(Strike Fire)
Symbolism: Military
Prowess, Bravery,
Manhood Status, Cause
and Effect.

**47. OHENE KRA
KONMUDE**
(Triangular Royal Pendant)
Symbolism: Three sources
(God, Ancestral Spirits and
the People) Spiritual Au-
thority, Protection of the
King, Sanctity and Divinity
of Royal Leadership.

43. AKOFENA
(State Ceremonial
Swords)
Symbolism: Balance
of Power, Political and
Legal Authority, Legiti-
macy Oath of Allegiance
and Political Loyalty.

**48. OHENE KRA
KONMUDE**
A version of (No.47)
(Royal Soul Pendant)
Symbolism: The king wears
this gold or silver pendant
when sitting in state during
special occasions.

44. AKOBEN
(War Horn)
Symbolism: Call to
collective action, Valor,
Military Readiness,
Spirit or Volunteerism
and Unity of Action.

**49. OHENE KRA
KONMUNDE**
(Circular Royal Soulful
Pendant) Another version.
Symbolism: Wholeness
and Sanctity of the Power
of the King rooted in the
infinite and Divine Power
of God.

45. AKOBEN
A version of (No. 44)
Other symbolism:
Collective Work and
Responsibility, Political
Vigilance and Social
Mobilization.

50. OHENE TUO
(The King's Rifle)
Symbolism: Military
Leadership o f the King,
Military Prowess, Bravery,
Readiness and Gallantry.
Attainment of Manhood.

MAN-MADE OBJECTS

51. DUA AFE
(Wooden Comb)
Symbolism: Feminine Essence of Life, Love, Caring, Patience and Nurturing. Also Inner and Outward Beauty, Good Health Habits and Body Grooming.

52. KONSON-KONSON
(A Chain)
Symbolism: Unity, Interdependence, Cooperation, Family Links, Collective Responsibility.

53. TABONO
(Oars)
Symbolism: Industriousness, Confidence Forward Looking, Persistence and Determination

54. AGYIN DAWURU
(A gong belonging to Agyin, a faithful servant of the King)
Symbolism: Faithfulness, Loyalty, Dutifulness, Service and Call to Action.

55. DAME DAME
(Multiple alternated squares of the checker board game) Symbolism: Strategic thinking and action, High Intelligence, Wisdom, Balance in all life situations.
.

MAN-MADE OBJECTS

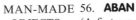

56. ABAN
(A fortress or a story house, also the seat of government)
Symbolism: Social Security, Centralized Political Authority, Power, Wealth, Prosperity and Superior Quality.

57. FI-HANKRA
(Enclosed and secured compound house)
Symbolism: Spiritual Protection, Social Security and Family Solidarity.

58. ABAN
(A fortress or a story house)
Symbolism: Seat of Government, Centralized Political System and Power, Fortitude, State Authority Magnificence.

Non-Figurative Shapes

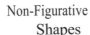

59. GYE NYAME
(Except God)
Symbolism: Such attributes of God as Omnipotence, Omniscience Omnipresence.

60. HYE WO NHYE
(Burn but won't burn)
Symbolism: Toughness, Imperishability, Endurance, Permanence of the essence of an individual or the King.

Non-Figurative Shapes

61. NKYIMKYIN
(Twistings)
Symbolism: Versatility
Adaptability, Dynamism,
Service, Balance in Life;
Ability to withstand
hardship and adjustto
changing life situations.

62. KRA PA or MUSYIDE
(Good Fortune Object for
Sanctification)
Symbolism: Sanctity of
the Soul. Good Fortune,
Spiritual Cleansing and
Spiritual Protection.

63. HWEHWEMUDUA
(Searching or Measuring
Rod)
Symbolism: Excellence,
Perfection, Refinement,
Knowledge, Superior
quality.

64. KRAMO BONE
(The Bad Moslem)
Symbolism: Warning
against deception,
hypocrisy and preten-
tiousness. Search for
genuiness and truth.

65. KRAMO BONE
A version of (No. 64)
The bad Moslem has made
it difficult for the good one
to be noticed.

Non-Figurative Shapes

66. SUNSUM
(The Soul)
Symbolism: Spiritual
Purity and Sanctity
of the Soul.

67. AWURADE NYANKOPON
(Mother/Father God)
Symbolism: Female
and Male Essences of the
Supreme Creator and
Creation itself.

68. AWURADE BAATANFO
(God the Mother)
Symbolism: Female
Attributes of the Divine
Creator, Mother-God,
the Motherness of the
Supreme One.

69. PEMPAMSIE
(Prepare for any action)
Symbolism: Readiness,
Steadfastness, Valor
Indestructible.

70. **KRONTI NE AKWAMU**
(Two compliment
ary branches of state)
Symbolism: Democratic
Principles, Balance of
Power, Duality of the
Essence of Life.

Non-Figurative Shapes

71. KUNTUN-KANTAN
(Inflated pride)
Symbolism: Warning against arrogance, pride extravagance and pomposity.

Non-Figurative Shapes

76. MATE MASIE
A version of (No. 75)
Symbolism: Readiness to Learn, Obedience and Thoughtfulness.

72. NYINSEN KRONKRON
(Divine Conception)
Symbolism: Sanctity & Divinity of Conception, Procreation, Fertility, Motherhood, Spiritual bond between parents and offsprings.

77. MRAMMUO
(Crossing)
Symbolism: Realities of Life's Challenges also Balance in Life, Reciprocity and Tolerance.

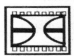

73. OBRA APUE NE NATOE
(Dawn and Dusk of Life)
Symbolism: Mutual Support between the old and the young: Longevity, Respect for elders.

78. ADINKRA HENE
(King of the Adinkra Symbols)
Symbolism: Greatness, Superior Quality, Firrmness, Magnanimity, Divinity of Creation.

74. OBAATAN PA
(The Good Mother)
Symbolism: Sanctity of Conception and Procreation and Motherhood.

79. ADINKRA HENE
A version of (No. 78)
Symbolism: Supremacy, and the Omnipotence of the Divine Creator and Creation itself; also Wholeness, Completeness and Superior Quality.

75. MATE MASIE
(I have kept what I have heard)
Symbolism: Wisdom, Knowledge, Prudence, Thoughtfulness.

80. AWARE PA
(Good Marriage)
Symbolism: Sanctity of Marriage, Patience, Devotion and Love.

Non-Figurative Shapes

81. DUA PA FRO
(Climbing a good tree)
Symbolism:
Encouragement,
Recognition of a good deed,
Assistance and
Incentive.

Non-Figurative Shapes

86. KOSAN
(Go and return or a Zigzag)
Symbolism: Balance in Life. Prudence and Perseverance.

82. DUA PA FRO
(Climbing a good tree)
Symbolism: Encouragement, Recognition of a good deed, Assistance and Incentive.

87. OSUA HU
(Learning to gain Knowledge)
Symbolism:
Knowledge, Wisdom, Experience and Intellectual Inquiry.

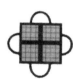

83. ABUSUA PA
(Good Family)
Symbolism: Family Unity, Family Links and Kinship ties.

CELESTIAL BODIES

88. OSRAM NE NSOROMMA
(Moon and Star)
Symbolism:
Faithfulness, Love, Loyalty, Harmony Fondness, Benevolence and Feminine Essence of life.

84. ABUSUA TE SE KWAAE
(The family is like a forest)
Symbolism: Unity in Diversity, Collectivity and Communality.

89. OSRAM
(Moon)
Symbolism: Faith, Patience and Determination.

85. NKYINKYIME
(Twistings)
Symbolism: Balance in life, Prudence and Perseverance.

90. NSOROMMA
(Star)
Symbolism: Faith, Loyalty, Greatness rooted in Allegiance to the Divine Power.

CELESTIAL
BODIES

91. OWIA KOKROKO
(Cosmic energy of the sun)
Symbolism: Vitality, Renewal, Procreative, Energy, Cosmic Energy, Growth and Enlightenment.

92. OWIA AHOODEN
(Life giving power of the sun)
Symbolism:
As in (No 91) God has a reason for keeping the sun at a distance.

93. DAB ME NSOROMA BEPUE
(My star will shine one day)
Symbolism: Hope, Faith, Aspiration Expectation and Confidence.

94. ASASE YE DURU
(The Earth is heavy)
Symbolism: Providence, the Divinity and Sanctity of Mother Earth, Procreation and Divine Source of Life's Sustenance.

95. ABODE SANTEN
(Eternity of Creation)
Symbolism: Eternity and Divinity of the Creation and the Creator.

PLANT
LIFE

96. DUA KRO
(Lone tree)
Symbolism: Need for cooperation, Interdependence Family Unity and Warning against Selfishness.

97. BESE SAKA
(Bunch of Cola Nuts)
Symbolism: Affluence Power, Abundance and Unity.

98. NKRUMAKESE
(The Big Okra)
Symbolism: Greatness, Superior quality and Wisdom.

99. NYAME DUA
(God's tree or God's altar)
Symbolism: The presence of God and his protection, Sacredness. Reverence to the Supreme Being and the Ancestors.

100. WAWA ABA
(Seed of the Wawa Tree)
Symbolism: Endurance, Hardiness, Persistence and Perseverance.

PLANT
LIFE

101. **AYA**
(Fern)
Symbolism: Endurance,
Perseverance, Independence
and Resourcefulness;
Peaceful Coexistence and
Mutual adaptability.

102. **NYAME NTI**
(Since God exists)
Symbolism: Faith, Hope
and Trust in God.

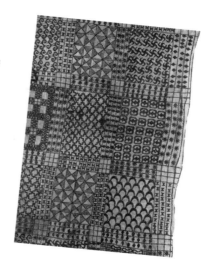

Example of an **Adinkra Cloth**

103. **FOFO**
(Seeds of the fofo plant).
Symbolism: Warning
against jealousy, hatred
and covetousness.

The information and designs on the Adinkra Symbols were
researched, written and designed by Dr. Kwaku Ofori Ansa,
Associate Professor of African Art History at Howard
University in Washington, D.C.

If you are interested in purchasing a 20 x 30 color poster
that includes a full description of the symbols please contact:

Sankofa Edu - Cultural Publications
2211 Amherst Road
Hyattsville, Maryland 20783
Phone 301-422-1821
Fax 301-422-0130
* Volume discounts available

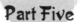

Part Five

HIV/AIDS

Nationwide Resource Listings

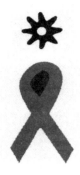

Here is a resource list of agencies and organizations located around the country that provide healthcare information and services on HIV/AIDS prevention, testing, peer counseling, emergency assistance, substance abuse and other social programs. (For more information check with your doctor or local health care provider.)

NATIONAL HOTLINES

Centers for Disease Control and Prevention (CDC) National AIDS Hotline
1-800-342-AIDS
(To get the Hotline # for your state visit)
www.cdc.gov

AIDS-INFO
1-800-HIV-0440
www.aidsinfo.nih.gov

National AIDS Hispanic Hotline
1-800-344-7432

National Pediatric HIV Resource Center
1-800-362-0071
www.pedhivaids.org

NATIONAL ORGANIZATIONS

African American Prevention Intervention Network
1-866-578-6872 (Jackson, MS)
www.ainonline.org

AID for AIDS / AFRICA
510-839-2241 (Oakland, CA)
www.aidforaidsafrica.org

AIDS Action Council (AAC)
202-530-8030 (Washington, DC)
www.aidsaction.org

AIDS Alliance for Children, Youth and Families
202-785-3564 (Washington, DC)
www.aids-alliance.org

American Red Cross
National AIDS Education Office
703-206-6000 (Washington DC)
www.redcross.org

Black Aids Institute
213-353-3610 (Los Angeles, CA)
www.blackaids.org

Center for AIDS Prevention Studies (CAPS)
415-507-9100 (San Francisco, CA)
www.caps.ucsf.edu

Center For Disease Control & Prevention
www.cdc.gov

Mississippi Urban Research Center
601-979-4193 (Jackson, MS)
www.murc.org

Moorhouse School of Medicine Aids Research Consortium
404-752-1706 (Atlanta, GA)

National AIDS Education and Services for Minorities
1-877-974-2376 (Atlanta, GA)

www.naesmonline.com

National Association of People with AIDS
202-898-0414   (Washington, DC)
www.napwa.org

National Black Man's Health Network
404-524-7237   (Atlanta, GA)

National Black Women's Health Projects (NBWHP)
202-543-9311   (Washington, DC)
www.nbwhp.org

National Black Leadership Commission on AIDS   (NBLCA)
212-614-0023   (New York, NY)
www.nblca.org

National Latina Health Network
202-965-9633   (New York, NY)
www.nationallatinahealthnetwork.com

National Minority AIDS Council
202-483-6622   (Washington, DC)
www.nmac.org

National Network for Youth
202-783-2949   (Washington, DC)
nn4youth@worldnet.att.net

National Organization of Concerned Black Men Inc.
202-783-6119   (Washington, DC)
www.cbmnational.org

National Prison Project   (NPP)
202-393-4930   (Washington, DC)

National United Church of HIV/ AIDS Network
216-736-2100   (Cleveland, OH)

National Youth Advocacy Coalition

202-319-7596   (Washington, DC)
www.nyacyouth.org

Philadelphia Figjht
215-985-4851   (Philadelphia, PA)
www.critpath.org

Planned Parenthood Federation of America
1-800-230-7526
www.plannedparenthood.org

The Balm In Gilead
212-730-7381   (New York, NY)
www.balmingilead.org

CHURCHES & SPIRITUAL SUPPORT

AIDS Ministry Network of the Christian Church
517-355-9324   (East Lansing, MI)
www.aidsfaith.com

AIDS National Interfaith Network
202-842-0010   (Washington, DC)
www.thebody.com/anin/aninpage

Allen Temple
510-544-8910   (Oakland, CA)
www.allen-temple.org

Antioch Baptist Church
216-791-0638   (Cleveland, OH)

Baptist AIDS Partnership
919-554-3220   (Wake Forest, NC)
www.baptistaidspartnership.org

Berean Missionary Baptist Church
718-774-0466   (Brooklyn, NY)
www.bereanbaptist.org

Buddhist AIDS Project (BAP)
415-522-7473   (San Francisco, CA)

www.buddhistaidsproject.org

Christian Faith Baptist Church
919-833-5834   (Raleigh, NC)
www.cfbc-ral.org

Church of the Living God Ministries
865-540-8767   (Knoxville, TN)

Dignity USA
1-800-877-8797 (Washington, DC)
www.dignityusa.org

Downs AME Church
510-654-5858

Emmanuel Seventh Day Adventist Church
251-479-1215   (Mobile, AL)

Eternal Life Christian Center
732-846-9153   (Somerset, NJ)
www.elcc.net

Faith Baptist Church
631-732-1133   (Coram, NY)
www.faithbaptist2.org

Faith Deliverance Christian Center
757-624-1900   (Norfolk, VA)

Friendship West Baptist Church
214-371-0964   (Dallas, TX)
www.friendshipwest.org

Glide-Goodlett HIV/AIDS Project
415-771-6300   (San Francisco, CA)
www.glide.org

Graham AME Church
843-766-0084   (Charleston, SC)
www.amec.org

Harlem Congregation for Community
Improvement   (HCCI)
212-283-5266   (New York, NY)
www.harlemcongregation@msn.com

Health Force Community Prevention
Health Institute
718-585-8585   (Bronx, NY)
healthforce@netzero.net

Historic Charles Street AME Church
617-442-7770   (Roxburg, MS)
www.csame.org

Holy Spirit Healing Ministry
816-763-4187   (Kansas City, MO)
anyanwu9@msn.com

Holy Temple Christian Center
401-861-9739   (Providence, RI)

Innerlight Unity Fellowship Church
202-544-7988   (Washington, DC)
www.ufcnc.org

Lutheran AIDS Network
609-396-4071   (Trenton, NJ)
www.lutheranservices.org

Memorial Baptist Church
212-663-8830   (New York, NY)
www.mbcvision2000@aol.com

Metropolitain Interdenominational
Church
615-726-3876   (Nashville, TN)
www.metropolitanfrc.com

Mt. Olivet Baptist Church
651-227-4444   (St. Paul, MN)

Mt. Sinai United Christian Church
718-447-8389   (Staten Island, NY)

National Catholic AIDS Network
707-874-3031   (Sebastopol, CA)
www.ncan.org

National Episcopal AIDS Coalition
718-857-9445   (Brooklyn, NY)

National United Church HIV/AIDS

Network
216-736-2100 (Cleveland, OH)

Presbyterian AIDS Network
412-330-4169

Shiloh Abundant Life Center
301-735-5100 (Forestville, MD)

St. John's United Methodist Center
713-659-3237 (Houston, TX)

St. Philip's Church
212-862-4940 (New York, NY)
www.stphilips-harlem.org

The Balm in Gilead
212-730-7381 (New York, NY)
www.balmingilead.org

United Church of Christ
216-736-3708 (Cleveland, OH)

United Methodist HIV/AIDS Ministries
Network
212-870-3870 (New York, NY)
www.gbgm-umc.org

Unity Fellowships Church Movement
866-227-4512 (Los Angeles, CA)
www.ufc-usa.org

Universal Fellowship of Metropolitan
Community Churches
310-360-8640 (West Hollywood, CA)
www.mcchurch.org

University Park Baptist Church
704-392-1681 (Charlotte, NC)

Wesley Chapel United Methodist Church
843-394-8458 (Lake City, SC)

Wider Church Ministries
(United Church of Christ)
216-736-3217 (Cleveland, OH)
www.ucc.org

OTHER ORGANIZATIONS and STATE HOTLINES

Alabama
State Hotline   1-800-228-0469
                 334-506-5634

AIDS Alabama
205-324-9822 (Birmingham)
www.aidsalabama.org

AIDS Services Center
256-832-0100 (Anniston)

Anchor
334-793-5709 (Dothan)
www.wiregrasspartnership.com

Birmingham AIDS Outreach
205-322-4197 (Birmingham)
www.aidsalabama.org

Birmingham Health Care for the
Homeless
205-212-5600 (Birmingham)
www.birminghamhealthcare.org

Dallas County Health Department
334-874-2550 (Selma)
www.adph.org

Davis Clinic
256-536-4700 (Huntsville)

DCH Regional Medical Center
205-759-7111 (Tuscaloosa)
www.dchsystem.com

Franklin Memorial Primary Health
Center
251-432-4117 (Mobile)

Houston County Health Department
334-793-1911 (Dothan)
www.adph.org

Jefferson County Aids in Minorities Inc.
205-781-1654   (Birmingham)

Madison County Health Department
256-539-3711   (Huntsville)

Mobile AIDS Support Services
251-471-5277   (Mobile)
www.masshelps.org

Mobile County Health
251-690-8832   (Mobile)

Montgomery AIDS Outreach
334-280-3388   (Montgomery)
www.mnv.net/mao

Montgomery County Health
Department
334-393-6400   (Montgomery)

Planned Parenthood
205-322-2121   (Birmingham)

Planned Parenthood
251-432-3211   (Mobile)

Talladega County Health Department
256-362-2593   (Talladega)

University of Alabama
Health Education and Wellness
205-348-3878   (Tuscaloosa)
www.ua.edu

University of Alabama at Birmingham
AIDS Center
205-934-2437   (Birmingham)
www.uabcfar.uab.edu

West Alabama AIDS Outreach
205-759-8470   (Tuscaloosa)
waao@bellsouth.net

Alaska
State Hotline   1-800-478-2437
                907-269-8000

Municipality of Anchorage Health
and Human Services
907-343-4611   (Anchorage)

Planned Parenthood
907-565-7526   (Anchorage)

STOP AIDS Project
907-278-5019   (Anchorage)
stopaids@ak.net

Arizona
State Hotline   1-800-334-1540
                602-230-5819

AIDS Project Arizona
602-253-2437   (Phoenix)
www.apaz.org

Arizona State University
Student Health and Wellness
480-965-3346   (Tempe)
www.asu.edu

Body Positive
602-307-5330   (Phoenix)
www.phoenixbodypositive.org

Insiders Program / Cope
520-798-1772   (Tuson)

Maricopa County Dept. of Public
Health
HIV Clinic
602-506-1678   (Phoenix)

McDowell Health Care Center
602-344-6550   (Phoenix)

Navajo AIDS Project
928-674-5676   (Chinle)
www.navahoaidsnetwork.org

Mujer- Sana
520-670-9075   (Tuscon)

The Ebony House

602-276-4288   (Phoenix)
ebonyhouse@quest.net

Together Responsibilities Informed
Black and Empowered   TRIBES
602-253-2457   (Phoenix)
www.apaz.org

Arkansas

State Hotline   1-800-482-5400
                 501-661-2408

Ark AIDS Foundation
501-376-6299   (Little Rock)
www.arkaidsfoundation.org

Arkansas Department of Health
501-661-2000   (Little Rock)

Arkansas Supportive Housing
Network
501-372-5543   (Little Rock)
www.ashn.org

Black Community Developer Inc.
501-663-9621   (Little Rock)
www.bcdinc.org

Centers for Youth & Families
501-666-9066   (Little Rock)

HIV/AIDS Center
479-452-1616   (Fort Smith)
www.fortsmithfightsaids.org

Planned Parenthood Center of
Arkansas and Eastern Oklahoma Inc.
501-666-7528   (Little Rock)

RAIN Arkansas
501-376-6090   (Little Rock)
www.rainark.org

The Women's Project
501-372-5113   (Little Rock)
www.womens-project.org

Washington County Health Department
HIV Clinic
479-973-8450   (Fayetteville)
www.washhealth.org

California

State Hotlines   1-415-863-2437
                  1-800-367-2437
www.aidshotline.org

AID for AIDS / AFRICA
510-839-2241   (Oakland)
www.aidforaidsafrica.org

AIDS/HIV Nightline
415-434-2437   (San Francisco)

AIDS Project East Bay
510-663-7979   (Oakland)
www.apeb.org

AIDS Project Los Angeles
213-201-1600   (Los Angeles)
www.apla.org.apeb.org

AIDS Resources Information Services
of Santa Clara Valley (ARIS)
408-293-2747   (San Jose)
www.aris.org

AIDS Service Foundation of Orange
County
949-253-1500   (Irvine)
www.ocasf.org

Alameda County African American
State of Emergency Task Force
510-874-7850   (Oakland)

Alameda County Public Health
Department Office of AIDS
510-873-6500   (Oakland)
www.alamada.ca.us/publichealth

Alameda Health Consortium
510-567-1550   (Oakland)

African-American Aids Services and
Survival Institute (AMASSI)
310-419-1969 (Englewood)
www.amassi.com

Ark of Refuge Inc.
415-861-1060 (San Francisco)
www.arkofrefuge.org

Ashay by the Bay
The Mindful Messages Mentoring Program
510-520-2742 (Union City)
www.ashaybythebay.com

Asian Health Services
510-986-6830 (Oakland)

Asian & Pacific Islander Wellness Center
415-292-3420 (San Francisco)
www.atiwellness.org

A Woman's Place
415-487-2140 (San Francisco)

Bay Area Black Consortium For Health Care
510-763-1872 (Oakland)

Bay Area Urban League
510-632-8285 (Oakland)

Bay Area Young Positives (BAY+)
415-487-1616 (San Francisco)
www.baypositive.org

Being Alive Center for Women and Children
619-291-1400 (San Diego)
www.beingalive.org

Berkeley Women's Health Center
510-843-6194 (Berkeley)

BLACK AIDS
213-353-3610 (Los Angeles)
www.blackaids.org

Black Coalition on AIDS Inc. (BCA)
415-615-9945 (San Francisco)

www.bcoa.org

Breaking Barriers
916-447-2437 (Sacramento)
www.breakingbarriers.org

California Dept. of Health and Human
Prevention Services Office of AIDS
916-445-0553 (Sacramento)
www.dhs.ca.goaids

CALPEP)
510-874-7850 (Oakland)
www.calpep.org

Catholic Charities of the East Bay
510-768-3100 (Oakland)
www.cceb.org

Center for AIDS, Research, Education
and Services (CARES)
916-443-3299 (Sacramento)
www.caresclinic.org

Children's Hospital of Los Angeles
Adolescent Medicine
323-669-2112 (Los Angeles)

Children's Hospital Oakland / Pediatric
AIDS/HIV Program
510-428-3010 (Oakland)
www.chofoundation.org/hospital

Circle of Care
510-531-7551 (Oakland)
www.ebac.org

City of Berkeley HHS AIDS Education
and Prevention
510-644-6355 (Berkeley)

City of Refuge
510-382-9166 (Oakland)
www.arkofrefuge.org

Contra Costa County Public Health
AIDS Program

925-313-6771　(Martinez)
www.co.contra-costa.ca.us

East Bay AIDS Center (EBAC)
510-204--1870　(Berkeley)
www.ebac.org

East Bay Community Law Center
510-548-4040　(Oakland)
www.ebclc.org

East Bay Community Recovery
510-446-7120　(Oakland)

Family Health Care Center
310-802-6177　(Redondo Beach)

Family Health Center of San Diego
619-515-2586　(San Diego)

First African Methodist Episcopal
Church (FAME)
323-737-0897　(Los Angeles)
www.firstame.org

Fresno County Health Services
HIV/AIDS Program
559-445-3569　(Fresno)
ww.fresnoca.gov

HEPPAC
510-547-0300　(Oakland)

Highland Hospital HIV Testing
510-437-8377　(Oakland)

Hollywood Clinic AIDS Healthcare
323-662-0196　(Los Angeles)

Hydeia L. Broadbent Foundation
323-874-0883　(Los Angeles)
www.hydeia.org

Iris Center
415-864-2364　(San Francisco)
www.citysearch.com/sfo/iriscenter

Kaiser Permanente/Santa Clara HIV/
AIDS Resource and Counseling
408-236-4170　(Santa Clara)

Kern County Health Department
AIDS Project
661-868-0360　(Bakersfield)
www.countyof kern.gov

La Clinca de La Raza
510-535-4155　(Oakland)

Laguna Beach Community Center
949-497-8473　(Laguna Beach)
www.lbcclinic.org

Laguna Shanti
949-494-1446　(Laguna Beach)
www.lagunashanti.org

Los Angeles County Dept. of Health
Office of AIDS (Programs and Policy)
213-351-8000　(Los Angeles)

Los Angeles Free Clinic
323-653-8622　(Los Angeles)
www.lafreeclinic.org

LYRIC
(For Lesbian, Gay, Bisexual,
Transgender and Questioning Youth)
414-703-6150　(San Francisco)
www.lyric.org

Magic Johnson Foundation
1-888-624-4205　(Culver City)
www.majicjohnson.org

Marin AIDS Project
415-457-2487　(San Rafael)
www.marinaidsproject.org

Minority AIDS Project
323-936-4949　(Los Angeles)
www.map.org

Monterey County Health Department
HIV/AIDS Prevention
831-647-7932   (Monterey)

National Native American AIDS
Prevention Center
510-444-2051   (Oakland)
www.nnaapc.org

New Connections Concord
925-363-5000   (Concord)
www.newconnections.com

Orange County AIDS Division AIDS
Information
714-834-8787   (Santa Ana)

PACE Clinic
408-885-5935   (San Jose)
www.hhs.co.santa-clara.ca.us

Planned Parenthood
925-754-4550   (Antioch)

Planned Parenthood of Central California
661-634-1000   (Bakersfield)

Planned Parenthood World Population
626-443-3878   (Los Angeles)

Planned Parenthood
209-579-2300   (Modesto)

Planned Parenthood
510-222-5290   (Richmond)

Planned Parenthood
805-963-2445   (Santa Barbara)

Planned Parenthood
925-838-2108   (San Ramon)

Planned Parenthood
831-758-8261   (Seaside)

Planned Parenthood
925-935-3010   (Walnut Creek)

Project Wise Women's Information
Service and Exchange
1-800-822-7422 (Hotline)
415-558-8669   (San Francisco)
www.projectinform.org

San Francisco AIDS Foundation
415-487-3000   (San Francisco)
www.sfaf.org

San Mateo County AIDS Program
650-573-3955   (San Mateo)
www.volunteerinfo.org/smcaids.htm

Santa Clara County AIDS Health
Services
408-494-7870   (San Jose)

Sexual Minority Alliance Alameda
County   (SMAAC)
510-834-9578   (Oakland)
www.smaac.org

St. Joseph's Medical Center
209-943-2000   (Stockton)
www.sjrhs.org

Tapestry
415-346-3512   (San Francisco)

The Center (Gay and Lesbian)
714-534-0961   (Orange County)
www.thecenteroc.org

The Clinic Inc.
323-295-6571   (Los Angeles)

The Earvin Magic Johnson Jr. Clinic
510-628--0949   (Oakland)

Tiburcio Vasquez Health Center
510-471-5907   (Union City)

Tracy Family Practice
209-820-1500   (Tracy)
www.cmc.com

Tri-City Health Center
510-713-6685   (Fremont)
510-727-9233   (Hayward)

UCLA Hospital and Medical Center
310-825-9146   (Los Angeles)
www.sectioncentral.md.ucla.edu

UCSD Med. Cnt. Pediatric Dept.
Mother, Child, Adolescent HIV
Program
619-298-2698   (San Diego)

United Black Men of Fresno
559-498-7701   (Fresno)
www.ubm.com

Watts Health Center
323-564-4331   (Los Angeles)

West Oakland Health Council Inc.
510-835-9610   (Oakland)
www.wohc.org

Westside Women's Health Clinc
310-450-2191   (Santa Monica)
www.wwhcenter.org

Women Alive UCLA Women
and Family Support
323-965-1564   (Los Angeles)
www.womenalive.org

Women Organized to Respond to Life
Threatening Diseases (WORLD)
510-986-0340   (Oakland)
www.womenhiv.org

Colorado

State Hotline   1-303-692-2777

AIDS Medicines and Miracles
303-860-8104   (Denver)

Boulder County AIDS Project
303-444-6121   (Boulder)
www.bcap.org

Colorado AIDS Project
303-837-1501   (Denver)
www.colaids.org

Denver Area Youth Services
303-698-2300   (Denver)
www.denveryouth.org./programs

Denver Department of Public Health
Infectious Diseases AIDS Clinic
303-436-7240   (Denver)

Horizon House
303-980-9604   (Denver)

Northern Colorado AIDS Project
970-484-4469   (Fort Collins)

People of Color Coalition Against Aids
(POCCAA)
303-321-7965   (Denver)

Rain Colorado
303-355-5665   (Denver)

University of Colorado
HIV/AIDS Care Program
303-372-8683   (Denver)

Connecticut

State Hotline   1-860--522-4636
                1-860-509-7800

AIDS Interfaith Network Inc.
203-624-4350   (New Haven)
aidsinterfaith@snet.net

AIDS Project Hartford
1-860-951-4833   (Hartford)
www.aidsprojecthartford.org

AIDS Project New Haven
203-624-0947   (New Haven)
www.uwgnh.org

Bridgeport Community Health Center
203-696-3260   (Bridgeport)

www.bridgeportchc.org

Connecticut Department of Health
1-860-509-7800 (Hartford)
www.state.ct.us

Human Resources Agency
1-860-826-4482 (New Britain)

New Haven Health Depot AIDS Div. 203-946-8707 (New Haven)

Delaware
State Hotline   1-800-422-0429
                 302-652-6776
 AIDS Delaware
302-652-6776 (Wilmington)
www.aidsdelaware.org

Catholic Charities
302-762-9244 (Wilmington)

District of Columbia
State Hotline   1-800-332-2437
                 202-727-2500

Abundant Life Clinic (A Muslim Clinic)
202-547-6440 (Washington, DC)
www.alclinic.org

AIDS Alliance for Children, Youth &
Families
202-785-3564 (Washington, DC)
www.aids-alliance.org

District of Columbia Dept. of Health
HIV/AIDS
202-727-2500 (Washington, DC)
www.dchealth..com

Family & Medical Counseling Services Inc.
202-889-7900 (Washington, DC)

George Washington University
GWU Medical Center
202-715-4000   (Washington, DC)
202-741-3000   Aids Clinic

www.gwdocs.com

HIV Community Coalition
202-543-6777 (Washington, DC)
www.hccmetrodc.org

Howard University Hospital HIV Clinic
202-865-1970 (Washington, DC)
www.howard.edu

Metro Teen Aids
202-543-9355 (Washington, DC)
www.metroteenaids.org

My Brother Keepers
202-806-4097 (Washington, DC)
www.mybrotherskeeperonline.org

Neighborhood Hunt Place Healthcare
202-388-8160 (Washington, DC)

Regional Addiction Prevention
202-462-7500 (Washington, DC)

Safe Haven Outreach Ministry Inc.
202-589-1505 (Washington, DC)
www.safehavenoutreach.org

Sasha Bruce Youthwork
202-675-9340 (Washington, DC)
www.sashabruce.org

Sexual Minority Youth Assistance
League (SMYAL)
202-546-5940 (Washington, DC)
202-546-5911   Helpline
www.smyal.org

Us Helping Us, People Into Living Inc.
202-546-8200 (Washington, DC)
www.ushelpingus.com

Washington Free Clinic
202-667-1106 (Washington, DC)
www.digitalfunk.com/freeclinic

Whitman-Walker Clinic Inc.

202-797-3500   (Washington DC)
www.wwc.org

Florida

State Hotline 1-800-224-6333 English
1-800-545-SIDA Spanish
1-800-243-7101 Haitian
1-850-224-6333 Inside

AIDS Oasis
850-314-0950   (Fort Walton)
www.aidoasis.org

AIDS Project Florida (APFL)
954-537-4111   (Ft. Lauderdale)
www.apfl.org

Broward House Inc.
954-522-4749   (Ft. Lauderdale)
www.browardhouse.org

Camillus Health Concern, Inc
305-757-9555   (Miami)

Catholic Charities Diocese of St.
Petersburg
813-631-4370

Center for Haitian Studies Inc.
305-757-9555
www.chsinfo@bellsouth.net

Comprehensive AIDS Program of
Palm Beach County (CAP)
561-844-1019   (Riviera)

Comprehensive AIDS Program CAP
561-687-3400   (Palm Beach)

Escambia AIDS Services
850-456-7079   (Pensacola)
ease3264@hotmail.com

Greater Bethel A.M.E. Church
305-379-8250   (Miami)
www.revmlusher@aol.com

Julius Adams AIDS Task Force, Inc.
(JAATA)
305-295-2437   (Key West)
jaatfinc@aol.com

Lock Towns Community Mental
Health
305-628-8981   (Miami)
www.locktowns.com

Martin Luther King Jr. Clinic With
Compensina HIV
305-342-6064   (Homestead)

Minorities Overcoming The Virus
Through Education (Movers Inc.)
305-754-7199   (Miami)

Mt. Pleasant Missionary Baptist
Church
407-841-3658   (Orlando)

Northwest Behavioral Health Services
904-781-7797   (Jacksonville)
www.nwbh.org

Northeast Florida AIDS Network
904-356-1612   (Jacksonville)
www.nfanjax.org

Operation Hope
727-822-2437   (St. Petersburg)
www.ohop.org

Planned Parenthood
954-561-1905   (Ft. Lauderdale)

Planned Parenthood
850-574-7455   (Tallahassee)

Planned Parenthood of Greater Miami
Clinic
305-285-5535   (Miami)

Shands Hospital at the University of
Florida
352-265-0110   (Gainesville)

www.shands.org

South Florida AIDS Network
305-585-5241   (Miami)

Tampa AIDS Network Florida Inc.
Womens AIDS Resource Movement
(WARM)
813-983-3333   (Tampa)

Tampa Hillsborough Action Plan Inc.
813-218-9021   (Tampa)

United Counties Minority AIDS Care and
Education
850-437-9000   (Pensacola)

University of Miami Aids Clinical
Research
305-243-3838   (Miami)
www.gate.net/-murc/

Work America, Inc.
305-576-8410   (Miami)
www.workamerica.org

Georgia
State Hotline   1-800-551-2728
                 404-876-9944
Aids Atlanta
404-870-7700   (Atlanta)
www.aidsatlanta.org

Aniz Inc.
New Life Support Center
404-758-1450   (Atlanta)
www.anizinc.org

Atlanta Interfaith Network
404-874-8686   (Atlanta)

Believe and Receive Ministry Inc.
404-294-0074   (Decature)
Center for Black Women's Wellness Inc.
404-688-9202   (Atlanta)

www.cbww.org

DeKalb Prevention Alliance
404-501-0722   (Decatur)
www.dekalballiance.org

Fulton County District and County
Health Department HIV/AIDS
404-730-1430   (Atlanta)

Jerusalem House Inc.
404-527-7627   (Atlanta)
www.jerusalemhouseinc.org

Our Common Welfare Inc.
404-297-9588   (Decature)
www.ourcommonwelfare.com

Outreach Inc.
404-755-6700   (Atlanta)
www.outreachincatlanta.org

Phoenix Project
912-231-0123   (Savannah)
www.unionmission.org

Planned Parenthood of Greater Atlanta
404-688- 9300   (Atlanta)
www.ppga.org

Project Azuka
912-233-6733   (Savannah)
www.azuka.org

Saint Joseph Mercy Care Services
404-880-3550   (Atlanta)
www.stjosephsatlanta.org

Sister Love Women's AIDS Project
404-753-7733   (Atlanta)
www.sisterlove.org

Hawaii
State Hotline   1-800-321-1555
                 808-733-9281

Planned Parenthood of Hawaii
808-589-1149 (Honolulu)

Maui AIDS Foundation
808-242-4900 (Wailuku)
www.mauiaids.org

Waikiki Health Center
808-922-4787 (Honolulu)

Idaho
State Hotline 1-800-926-2580
208-334-6527
Idaho AIDS Foundation
208-321-2777 (Boise)

Idaho Dept. of Health and Welfare
208-334-6527 (Boise)
www.2.state.id.us./dhw

Planned Parenthood Assoc. of Idaho
208-376-9300 (Boise)

Illinois
State Hotline 1-800-243-2437
217-524-5983

Access Community Health Network
773-257-5099 (Chicago)
www.acesscommunityhealth.org

AIDS Care Net (ACN)
815-968-5181 (Rockford)

AIDS Foundation of Chicago
312-922-2322 (Chicago)
www.aidschicago.org

AIDS Legal Council
312-427-8990 (Chicago)
www.aidslegal.com

Alternative AIDS Health Project
773-561-2800 (Chicago)

Aunt Martha's Youth Service Center c.
708-754-1044 (Chicago Heights)

www.auntmarthas.org

Better Existence with HIV (BEHIV)
847-475-2115 (Evanston)
www.behiv.org

Catholic Charities of Chicago
312-655-7000 (Chicago)
www.catholiccharities.org

Chicago Department of Public Health
312-747-9865 (Chicago)
www.ci.chi.il.us

Chicago Health Outreach Clinic
773-275-2060 (Chicago)

Chicago Women's Aids Project
773-271-2070 (Chicago)

Christie Clinic
217-366-1200 (Champaign)
www.christiclinic.com

Circle Family Care
773-379-1000 (Chicago)

Columbia Michael Reese Hospital and
Medical
312-791-3455 (Chicago)

Cook County Hospital
312-572-4740 (Chicago)
www.corecenter.org

Dekalb County Health
815-758-6673 (Dekalb)

Friends of People With AIDS
309-671-2144 (Peoria)
www.friendsofpwa.org

Garfield Counseling Center
773-533-0433 (Chicago)
jlbjulia@aol.com

Greater Chicago Committee

773-287-3263   (Chicago)
velani063@aol.com

Harbor Light Center
312-421-5753   (Chicago)
www.salarmychicago.org

Heartland Human Services
217-347-7179   (Effingham)
heartland@heartland.org

Illinois Department of Public Health
217-524-5983   (Springfield)

Interfaith House
773-533-6013   (Chicago)
www.interfaithhouse.org

Kankakee County Health
815-937-3560   (Bradley)

Midwestern Prevention Intervention
Center
773-568-6245   (Chicago)
www.apinonline.org

Open Door Clinic
847-695-1093   (Elgin)
www.opendoorclinic.org

Planned Parenthood of Greater Peoria
309-673-6911   (Peoria)

Roseland Christian Health Ministries
773-233-4100   (Chicago)
www.c-c-h-c.org

Serenity House
630-620-6616   (Addison)
www.serenityhouse.org

Southern Illinois School of Medicine
217-545-0181   (Springfield)
www.siumed.edu

South Side Help Center
773-445-5445   (Chicago)

www.southsidehelp.org

Springfield Department of Public
Health
217-789-2182   (Springfield)

Task Force Aids Prevention
312-986-0661   (Chicago)

Test Positive Aware Network
773-989-9400   (Chicago)
www.tpan.com

Urban Lifeline Family Support
Center
773-768-3536   (Chicago)

Vida/Sida
773-278-6737   (Chicago)
www.vidasida.org

Vital Bridges
708-386-3383   (Oakpark)

Westside Holistic Family Services
773-921-8777   (Chicago)

Youth Service Project
773-772-6270   (Chicago)

Indiana
State Hotline   1-800-848-2437
                 317-920-7755

AIDS Ministries AIDS Assistance
574-234-2870   (South Bend)
www/aidsministries.org

AIDS Resource Group
812-421-0059   (Evansville)
www.argonsite.com

AIDS Task Force
765-983-3425   (Richmond)

AIDS Task Force of Northeast
260-744-1144   (Ft. Wayne)

www.aidsfortwayne.org

Aliveness Project
219-548-0194   (Valparaiso)

Boys and Girls Clubs of Indianapolis
317-920-4700   (Indianapolis)
www.bgindy.org

Community Action of Greater
Indianapolis
317-396-1800   (Indianapolis)
www.cagi-in.org

Concord Community Center
317-637-4376   (Indianapolis)
www.concordindy.org

Disciples Homeland Mission
1-888-346-2631 (Indianapolis)
www.homelandministries.org

Ft. Wayne Women's Bureau
260-424-7977   (Ft. Wayne)
www.womensbureau.com

Indiana Ministry Health Coalition Inc.
317-926-4011   (Indianapolis)
www.imhc.org

Indiana State Department of Health
317-233-1325   (Indianapolis)
www.in.gov/isdh

Marion County Bellflower HIV Clinic
317-221-8307   (Indianapolis)
www.mcnd.com

Matthew 25 Clinic
260-426-3250   (Ft. Wayne)
www.the_league.org/matthew

Monroe County Health Department
812-349-2542   (Bloomington)
www.co.monroe.in.us

Peoples Health Center

317-633-7360   (Indianapolis)

Steuben County Health Department
260-668-1000   (Angola)

The Outreach Project
317-927-5151   (Indianapolis)

Iowa
State Hotline   1-800-445-2437
                515-244-6700

AIDS Project of Central Iowa
515-284-0245   (Des Moines)

Iowa Center For AIDS
319-338-2135   (Iowa City)
www.icare/ia.org

Iowa Department Public Health
515-281-5787   (Des Moines)
www.idph.state.ia.us

Johnson County AIDS Project
379-356-6038   (Iowa City)

Planned Parenthood of Iowa
515-280-7000   (Des Moines)

Rapids AIDS Project
319-393-9579   (Cedar Rapids)
1-800-445-2437
rap@grantwoodredcross.org

Kansas
State Hotline   1-877-526-2347
                785-296-6036

AIDS Council of Greater Kansas City
816-751-5166   (Kansas City)
www.kc-reach.org

Good Samaritan Project
816-561-8784   (Kansas City)
www.kc-reach.org/kc-organizations

Kansas City Free Health Clinic
816-753-5144   (Kansas City)
www.kcfree.org

Kansas Dept. of Health (HIV/STD)
785-296-6173   (Topeka)
www.kdat.ks.us.com

Topeka AIDS Project
785-232-3100   (Topeka)
www.topekaaidsproject.org

Wichita Community Clinical AIDS
Program
316-265-9468   (Wichita)
www.connectcareks.org

Kentucky
State Hotline   1-800-840-2865
                 502-564-6539

Center for Women and Families
502-581-7273   (Louisville)
www.thecenteronline.org

Glade House
502-587-5010   (Louisville)

Life Preserver
502-458-9319   (Louisville)

Louisville Jefferson County Aids Program
502-585-4733   (Louisville)
www.licolnfdn.org

Planned Parenthood
859-252-8494   (Lexington)

University of Kentucky Hospital
859-323-5000   (Lexington)
www.ukcc.uky.edu/cgi-bio.com

Louisiana
State Hotline   1-877-662-4371
                 504-821-2601

AIDS Minority Community Outreach

318-226-8717   (Shreeveport)

Brotherhood Incorporated
504-947-4100   (New Orleans)
www.brotherhoodinc.org

Children's Hospital Pediatric AIDS
Program
504-821-4611   (New Orleans)

Excelth Inc.
504-524-1210   (New Orleans)
www.excelth.com

Faces Program
504-821-4611   (New Orleans)

Friends for Life
225-923-2277   (Baton Rouge)
www.friendsforlifebr.org

Greater Ouachita Coalition for AIDS
318-325-1092   (Monroe)

Great Expectations Foundation Inc.
504-598-2229   (New Orleans)
www.greatexpectations.org

Louisiana Department of Health HIV
Program
504-568-7524   (Baton Rouge)
www.dhh.state.la.us

National Council of Negro Women
of Greater New Orleans
504-525-0798   (New Orleans)

Natural Resources for Preparing,
Education And Changing Environments
(N'R' Peace)
504-948-3537   (New Orleans)

New Orleans AIDS Task Force
504-821-2601   (New Orleans)
www.crescentcity.com/noaids/

Philadelphia Center

318-222-6633   (Shreeveport)
www.philadelphiacenter.org

South Roman Street Clinic
and Medical Center
504-903-7041   (New Orleans)

Velocity Foundation
504-486-2650   (New Orleans)
www.dhh.state.la.us

Maine
State Hotline   1-800-851-2437
                      207-774-6877
AIDS Project
207-774-6877   (Portland)
www.aidsproject.org

Coastal AIDS Network
207-338-6330   (Bellfast)
www.coastalaidsnetwork.org

Dayspring AIDS Support Network
202-621-6201   (Augusta)
www.healthreach.org

Downeat AIDS Network
207-667-3506   (Ellsworth)
www.downeat.net

Eastern Maine AIDS Network
207-990-3626   (Bangor)
www.maineaidsnetwork.com

The AIDS Project (TAP)
207-774-6877   (Portland)
www.maineaidsinfo.org

The Maine AIDS Alliance
The Main Department of Health
207-287-2747   (Augusta)

Maryland
State Hotline   1-800-638-6252 English
                      1-800-358-9001
                      410-767-5013

Baltimore Prevention Coalition
410-383-2800   (Baltimore)
www.baltimorepreventioncoalition.org

Baltimore Urban League
410-523-8150   (Baltimore)
www.bul.org

Baltimore Youth Services Bureau
410-276-1100   (Baltimore)

Black Women's Health Council Inc.
(BWHC)
301-772-3999   (Largo)
www.bwhc.info.org

Community Services Coalition
301-925-9280   (Largo/Landover)
cscpgc@smart.net

Ecumerial AIDS Resource Services Inc.
(EARS)
410-947-0700   (Baltimore)
bgt5161@aol.com

HIV/AIDS Volunteer Enrichment
Network (HAVEN Inc.)
410-224-AIDS   (Annapolis)
www.haven.inc.org

Johns Hopkins AIDS Services
1-800-765-JHHS
410-955-9444   (Baltimore)
www.hopkins-aids.edu

Maryland Department of Health
410-767-6535   (Baltimore)

Northwest Baltimore Corporation
410-542-6610   (Baltimore)
www.nwbcorp.org

Richard Allen Community
Development Corporation
301-583-0891   (Largo)
dspencer@capu.net

Sacred Zion Church / Project Arise
410-837-8400   (Baltimore)
www.sacredzion.org

Sisters Together And Reaching (STAR)
410-383-1903   (Baltimore)
debbie7rev@aol.com

Massachusetts
State Hotline   1-800-235-2331
                 617-536-7733

AIDS Action Committee
1-800-235-2331   (Boston)
www.aac.org

AIDS Project Worcester
508-735-3773   (Worcester)
www.aidsprojectworcester.org

Between Family and Friends
413-747-8236   (Springfield)

Cambridge Cares About AIDS
617-661-3040   (Cambridge)
www.ccaa.org

Greater Cambridge Health Alliance
617-665-1000   (Cambridge)

Moses Saunders AIDS Outreach Center
617-880-7950   (Dorchester)

Multicultural AIDS Coalition Inc.
617-442-1622   (Boston)
www.mac.boston.org

We Are Education With A Touch
(WEATOC)
617-541-5858   (Dorchester)
www.weatoc.com

Who Touched Me Ministry / AIDS
Action Community
617-450-1000   (Boston)
www.aac.org

Michigan
State Hotline   1-800-872-2437 English
                 313-446-9800

AIDS Partnerships Michigan
313-446-9800   (Detroit)
www.aidspartnership.org

Black Family Development
313-272-3500   (Detroit)
www.blackfamilydevelopment.org

Children's Immune Disorders
313-837-7800   (Detroit)
www.comnet.org/kids/index

Community AIDS Resource Service
(CARES)
269-381-2437   (Kalamazoo)
www.caresswm.org

Community Health Awareness Group
313-872-2424   (Detroit)

Community Health Outreach Workers
313-963-3352   (Detroit)

Detroit Unity Association
D. A. Brody Associates
313-927-0987   (Detroit)

HIV/AIDS Resource Centre
734-572-9355   (Ypsilanti)
www.rzhark.org

Men of Color Play It Safe (MOC)
313-543-7000   (Detroit)

Michigan Department of Community
Health
517-241-5933   (Lansing)
www.mdch.state.mi.us

Midwest AIDS Prevention
248-545-1435   (Ferndale)
www.aidsprevention.org

Planned Parenthood
734-973-0710   (Ann Arbor)

Planned Parenthood
810-234-1659   (Flint)

Planned Parenthood
616-372-1205   (Kalamazoo)
Project Survival
313-961-2027   (Detroit)

Sisters & Daughters of Sheba
313-927-3180   (Detroit)
www.sadosi.org

Wellness AIDS Services
810-232-0888   (Flint)

Minnesota
State Hotline   1-800-248-2437
                 612-373-2437

African American AIDS Task Force
612-825-2052   (Minneapolis)
www.aaataskforce@quest .net

City Inc.
612-724-3689   (Minneapolis)
www.cityinc.org

Community Fitness Today
612-824-8610   (Minneapolis)

Mayo HIV Clinic
507-255-7763   (Rochester)
www.mayo.org

Minneapolis Urban League
612-302-3100   (Minneapolis)
www.mul.org

Minnesota AIDS Project
612-341-2060   (Minneapolis)
www.mul.org

Minnesota Department of Human
Services HIV/AIDS Program

1-800-657-3761 (St. Paul)
www.dhss.state.mn.us

Missoula AIDS Council
406-543-4770   (Missoula)

Red Door Clinic
612-348-6363   (Minneapolis)
www.co.hennepin.mn.us/commhlth/
reddoor

Room 111
651-266-1352   (St. Paul)

The Aliveness Project
612-822-7946   (Minneapolis)
www.aliveness.org

Turning Point
612-520-4004   (Minneapolis)
www.ourturningpoint.org

Youth Intervention Project
612-348-3307   (Minneapolis)

Youth Link
612-252-1200   (Minneapolis)

University of Minnesota Youth and
AIDS Projects
612-627-6820   (Minneapolis)
www.yapmn.com

Mississippi
State Hotline   1-800-826-2961
                 601-576-7723

Adams County Health Department
601-445-4601   (Natchez)
www.msdh.state.ms.us

Building Bridges Inc.
601-922-0100   (Jackson)

5 Points Clinic
601-987-6728   (Jackson)

De Porres Health Center
662-326-9232   (Marks)

Improving Quality of Life
601-969-3733   (Jackson)

Jackson State University (MURC)
Mississippi Urban Research Center
601-979-4081   (Jackson)
www.jsums.edu

Jefferson County Health Department
228-762-1117   (Fayette)

New Life Ministry Inc./ Not Here
Foundation.
601-376-0707   (Jackson)
www.notherefoundation.org

Our House Inc.
662-334-6873   (Greenville)

South Mississippi AidsTask Force
228-385-1214   (Biloxi)
smatf@aol.com

The Rapp Team
Mississippi Children's Home Society
601-352-7784   (Jackson)
www.mchsfsa.org

University of Mississippi
601-984-1600   (Jackson)
www.demiss.edu

Warren County HIV/AIDS Services
807 Clinic
601-636-4356   (Vicksburg)

Missouri
State Hotline   1-800-533-2437
                  513-751-6141

Aids Council of Greater Kansas City
816-751-5166   (Kansas City)
www.kc-reach.org

AIDS Project of the Ozarks
417-881-1900   (Springfield)
www.aidsprojectoftheozarks.org

Black Health Care Coalition
816-444-9600   (Kansas City)
www.blackhealthcoalition.com

Blacks Assisting Blacks Against Aids
(BABAA)
314-865-1600   (St. Louis)
www.babaa.org

Catholic Charities
816-254-4100   (Independence)

Catholic Charities
816-221-4377   (Kansas City)

Cole County Health Department
573-636-2181   (Jefferson County)
www.colehealth.org/hiv-aids

Kansas City Free Health Clinic
816-753-5144   (Kansas City)
www.kcfree.org

Metropolitain Center HIV/AIDS Services
314-612-5188   (St. Louis)

Planned Parenthood
314-921-4445   (Florissant)

Regional Aids Interfaith Network (RAIN)
1-800-785-2437 (Columbia)
www.missourirain.com

St. Louis Effort for AIDS
314-645-6451   (Kansas City)
www.stlefa.org

University of Missouri Student Health
Center
573-882-7481   (Columbia)
www.hsc.missouri.edu

Montana

State Hotline   1-800-233-6668
                406-444-3565

Family Service Inc.
406-259-2269   (Billings)

Gallaten Country Health Department
406-582-3100   (Bozeman)
www.co.gallaten.net.us/health

Montana Department of Public Health
Human Services
406-444-5622   (Helena)

Nebraska

State Hotline   1-800-782-2437
                402-552-9255

Charles Drew Health Center/American
Red Cross
404-343-7700   (Omaha)

Nebraska AIDS Project
402-476-7000   (Lincoln)

Nebraska AIDS Project
402-552-9260   (Omaha)
www.nap.org

Nebraska Health and Human Services
402-471-2937   (Lincoln)
www.hhs.state.ne.us/std

Planned Parenthood
402-554-1045   (Omaha)

Nevada

State Hotline   1-775-684-5900

AID for AIDS in Nevada (AFAN)
702-382-2326   (Las Vegas)
www.insideafan.org

AIDS Community Cultural Education
Program and Training (ACCEPT)
775-348-2050   (Reno)

www.acceptreno.org

Clark County Health District
702-385-1291   (Las Vegas)
www.cchd.org

Northern Nevada Hopes
775-786-4673   (Reno)
www.med.nunr.edu-whinn-hopes

Planned Parenthood
702-878-3622   (Las Vegas)

The AIDS Drug Assistance Program
(ADAPT)
775-684-5952   (Carson City)

UMC Wellness Center
702-383-2691   (Las Vegas)
www.universitymedicalctr.com

New Hampshire

State Hotline   1-800-752-2437
                603-271-4502
Hope Clinic
775-786-4673   (Reno)

Planned Parenthood of Northern
New England
603-669-7321   (Bedford Hts.)

Southern New Hampshire HIV/AIDS
Task Force
603-595-8464   (Nashua)
info@aidstask.nh.org

New Jersey

State Hotline   1-800-624-2377

Catholic Charities
856-764-6945   (Delanco)

Faith Services / Office of AIDS
201-792-6161   (Hoboken)

Henry J. Austin Health Center
609-278-5946   (Trenton)

www.henryjaustin.org

Horizon Health Center
201-451-6300   (Jersey City)
www.horizonhealth.org

Hyacinth AIDS Foundation
973-565-0300   (Newark)

Hyacinth AIDS Foundation
732-246-0204   (New Brunswick)

Hyacinth AIDS Foundation
201-432-1134   (Jersey)
908-755-0021   (N. Plainfield)
973-278-7636   (Patterson)
609-396-8322   (Trenton)
www.hyacinth.org

Infoline of Middlesex County of New
Brunswick
732-418-0200   (New Brunswick)
www.info-line.org

Isaiah House
973-677-1530   (East Orange)
litufc@aol.com

Liberation in Truth Unity Fellowship
973-621-2100   (Newark)
www.members.aol.com/litanity

Newark Community Health Center
973-483-1300   (Newark)

New Jersey Div. of Disability Svcs. AIDS
Community Care Alternative Program
609-588-2620   (Trenton)
www.state.nj.us

New Jersey Division of AIDS
Prevention and Control
609-984-5894   (Trenton)
www.state.nj.us/health/

North Jersey AIDS Alliance
910-483-3444   (Newark)

Planned Parenthood Association of
Mercer County
609-599-4411   (Trenton)

Positive Health Care
973-596-9667   (Newark)
www.positive_healthcare.com

Rainbow House
609-394-6747   (Trenton)

South Jersey AIDS Alliance (ACCAP)
609-347-1085   (Trenton)
www.southjeseyaidsalliance.org

New Mexico
State Hotline   1-800-545-2437
                          505-476-3612

Agape African-American HIV Outreach
505-393-8787   (Hobbs)

New Mexico AIDS Services
505-938-7100   (Albuquerque)
www.nmas.net

New Mexico Department of Health
HIV/AIDS Prevention Services
505-476-3629   (Santa Fe)
www.health.state.am.us/websitesnsf

People of Color Aids Foundation
1-888-268-6579   (Santa Fe)
pocasofnm@cybermesa.com

Southwest Care Center
505-989-8200   (Santa Fe)

New York
State Hotline   1-800-872-2777 English
                          1-800-233-7431 Spanish
                          1-800-233-SIDA
Albany
                          716-845-3170

Adolescent AIDS Program Children's
Hospital of Montefiore
718-882-0232   (Bronx)
www.asolescentaids.org

African Services Committee Inc.
212-222-3882   (New York City)
www.africanservices.org

AIDS Community Services
716-847-2441   (Buffalo)
www.aidscommunityservices.com

AIDS Council of Northeast
518-434-4686   (Albany)
www.aidscouncil.org

AIDS Family Services
716-881-4612   (Buffalo)

AIDS Rochester Hotline
716-442-2200   (Rochester)

AIDS Treatment Data Network
1-800-734-7104 (New York)
www.aidstreat.org

Arthur Ashe Institute for Urban Health
718-270-3101   (Brooklyn)
www.arthurasheinstitute.org

Belleview Hospital Center AIDS
 Program
212-562-3906   (New York City)

Black Veterans
718-935-1116   (Brooklyn)

Body Positive
212-566-7333   (New York City)
www.bodypositive.com

Bronx Aid Services
718-295-5605   (Bronx)

Bronx Outreach Center
718-842-0870   (Bronx)

www.geocities.com

Brooklyn AIDS Task Force (BATF)
Williamsburg Health & Resource Center
718-622-2910   (New York City)
brandes@aol.com

Brownsville Community Development
Corporation
718-485-3820   (Brooklyn)

Caribbean Womens Health
718-940-8386   (Brooklyn)
www.cwha.org

Children's Hospital of Buffalo AIDS
Clinic
716-878-7000   (Buffalo)

Community Healthcare Network
Women's Center
718-991-9250   (New York City)
www.chnnyc.org

Group Ministries
716-883-4367   (Buffalo)

Haitian Center Council Inc.
718-855-7275   (Brooklyn)
www.haitiancentercouncil.org

Harlem Congregation for Community
Improvement (HCCI)
212-283-5266   (New York City)
www.hcci.org

Harlem Directors Group Inc.
212-531-0049   (New York City)
www.hdg.org

Harlem United Community AIDS
Center
212-531-1300   (New York City)
www.harlemunited.org

Hispanic AIDS Forum Inc.
212-563-4500   (Manhattan)

www.hafnyc.org

Interfaith Medical Center / Primary Clinic
718-935-7054   (Brooklyn)
kfingall@interfaithmedical.com

Iris House
212-423-9049   (New York City)
irishouse1@aol.com

Lenox Hill AIDS Center
212-434-2580   (New York City)

Life Force Women Fighting AIDS Inc.
718-797-0937   (Brooklyn)
lfwfainc@aol.com

Minority Task Force on AIDS
212-864-4046   (New York City)
www.minoritytaskforceonaids..org

Miracle Makers Inc.
718-483-3047   (Brooklyn)

Momentum AIDS Project
212-691-8100   (New York City)
www.momentumaidsproject.org

Mount Sinai Medical Center Adolescent
Health Center
212-423-3000   (New York City)

New York Department of Health AIDS
Initiatives
518-473-7542   (New York City)
www.ealt.state.ny.us

People of Color in Crisis
718-230-0770   (Brooklyn)
www.pocc.org

People With AIDS Coalition of New York
Sister to Sister Project
800-828-3280   (New York City)

Settlement Health
212-360-2600   (New York City)

www.settlementealt.org

The Door
212-941-9090   (New York City)

Vanguard Urban Improvement
Association Inc.
718-453-3330   (Brooklyn)
vuia3@erols.com

William F. Ryan Community Health
Center
212-316-7906   (New York City)

Womens Center
718-920-5157   (Bronx)

North Carolina

State Hotline   1-800-342-2437
                        919-733-3039
AIDS Aware
910-791-7598   (Wilmington)

AIDS Care Service (ACS)
336-777-0142   (Winston-Salem)
www.aidscareservice.org

Alliance of AIDS Services Carolina
(AASC)
919-596-9898   (Durham)
www.aas.c.org

Alliance of AIDS Services Carolina
(AASC)
919-834-2437   (Raleigh)

Cape Fear Regional Bureau
910-483-9177   (Fayetteville)
www.capefearinc.org

Cure AIDS of Wilmington
910-251-0744   (Wilmington)

Craven Regional Medical Center
252-633-8111   (New Bern)
www.cravenhealthcare.org

Duke University Medical Center
919-681 6261   (Durham)

Metrolina AIDS Project (MAP)
704-333-1435   (Charlotte)
www.metrolinaaidsproject.org

North Carolina Department of Health
HIV/AIDS Prevention and Care
919-733-7301   (Raleigh)
www.schs.state.nc.us./epi/hiv

Operation Sickle Cell Inc.
910-488-6118   (Fayetteville)
www.ancfsu.edu/osc

Regional AIDS Interfaith Network
(RAIN)
704-372-7246   (Charlotte)
www.carolinarain.org

Sickle Cell Disease Association of
Piedmont
336-274-1507   (Greensboro)
www.scdap.org

The Relatives
704-377-0602   (Charlotte)
www.youthnetworknc.org

Triad Health Project (THP)
336-275-1654   (Greensboro)
www.triadhealthproject.com

Wake Forest University
336-713-2000   (Winston-Salem)
www.bgsm.edu

Wake Teen Medical Services
919-828-0035   (Raleigh)

Whright Focus
336-454-5632   (Jamestown)
www.thedepot.com/groups-wright focus

North Dakota
State Hotline   1-800-706-3448
                 701-328-2378

Diocese of Bismarck
701-222-3035 (Bismarck)
www.bismarckdiocese.com

First Link
701-293-6462   (Fargo)

Merit Care
701-280-4100   (Fargo)
www.meritcare.com

Ohio
State Hotline   1-614-466-2144
                 614-332-2437

AIDS Resource Center - Ohio
937-461-2437   (Dayton)

AIDS Task Force of Greater Cleveland
216-621-0766 (Cleveland)
www.aidstaskforce.org

AIDS Volunteers
513-421-2437   (Cincinnati)
www.avoc.org

Athens AIDS Task Force
740-592-4397   (Athens)

Center for Families and Children
216-241-6400 (Cleveland)
www.community.cleveland.com

Children's Hospital Medical Center
513-636-4269   (Cincinnati)

Children's Medical Center
937-226-8300   (Dayton)

Cincinnati City Health Department
513-357-7350   (Cincinnati)

www.cincinnatihealth.org

Cleveland Free Clinic
216-721-4010   (Cleveland)
www.thefreeclinic.org

Columbus AIDS Task Force
614-299-2437   (Columbus)
www.catf.net

Community Action Against AIDS
Addiction
216-881-0765   (Cleveland)
caaraw@aol.com

Community AIDS Network
3375-2000   (Akron)

Crisis Center
530-452-6000   (Canton)

First Link
614-221-2255   (Columbus)

Health Wholeness Advocacy
216-736-2284   (Cleveland)
www.ucc.org

Howard Community Services
216-991-8585   (Cleveland)

Ohio Department of Health
614-466-3543   (Columbus)

Planned Parenthood of Southeast Ohio
740-593-3375   (Athens)

Planned Parenthood of Northeast Ohio
419-255-1123   (Toledo)

Stay AIDS Free Through Education
(SAFE)
216-991-7233   (Cleveland)
www.safe/.net

Toledo Lucas Health Department
STD Clinic

419-213-4100   (Toledo)

Violets Cupboard
330-375-2159   (Akron)
www.rainbowakron.com

Wider Church Ministries
216-736-3217   (Cleveland)
www.ctconfucc.org

Oklahoma
State Hotline   1-800-535-2437
                918-834-8378

Healing Hands
405-272-0476   (Oklahoma City)

Helpline
918-836-4357   (Tulsa)

Regional AIDS Interfaith Network
1-800-324-RAIN (Oklahoma City)

The Winds House
AIDS Support Program Inc.
405-525-6277   (Oklahoma City)
aspwwinds@aol.com

Tulsa Cares Consortium
918-834-4194   (Tulsa)
www.tulsacares.org

University of Children's Hospital of
Oklahoma Care Center
405-271-6208   (Oklahoma City)

Oregon
State Hotline   1-800-777-2437
                503-233-2437

Douglas County AIDS Council
1-877-440-2761 (Roseburg)
www.hivroseburg.org

HIV Alliance
541-342-5088   (Eugene)
www.hivalliance.org

Multnomah County Health Dept.
503-988-3030   (Portland)
www.co.multnomah.or.us

Oregon Department of Health
503-731-4029   (Portland)
www.state.or.us

Outside In
503-223-4121   (Portland)
www.outsidein.org

Planned Parenthood
541-344-2632   (Eugene)

Pennsylvania
State Hotline   1-800-662-6080
                 717-783-0573

Actions AIDS Center City
Winds House
215-981-0088   (Philadelphia)

Alpha House
412-363-4220   (Philadelphia)
www.alphahouseinc.org

Blacks Educating Blacks About Sexual
Health Issues
215-769-3561   (Philadelphia)

Catholic Charities
412-456-6999   (Pittsburgh)

Circle of Care
215-985-2657   (Philadelphia)
www.circleofcare.com

Concerned Black Men of Philadelphia
215-276-2806   (Philadelphia)
1-877-867-1446
www.cbmphilly.org

Pennsylvania Department of Health
Division of HIV/AIDS
717-783-0572   (Harrisburg)
www.health.state.pa.us

Philadelphia Fight
215-985-4448   (Philadelphia)
www.fight.org

Pittsburgh AIDS Task Force
412-242-2500   (Pittsburgh)
www.patf.org

The Philadelphia AIDS Consortium
215-988-9902   (Philadelphia)
www.tpaconline.org

The Phildelphia Alliance
215-438-6400   (Philadelphia)
www.philalliance.org

To Our Children's Future with Health
215-879-7740   (Philadelphia)

Germantown Settlement
215-545-6868   (Philadelphia)

Women with Immune System
Disorders. Org
215-991-6550   (Philadelphia)

Women's Christian Alliance
215-236-9911   (Philadelphia)
www.wcafamily.org

Youth Outreach Adolescent Awareness
Program/GPVAC
215-851-1846   (Philadelphia)
www.yoaap.org

Puerto Rico
State Hotline   1-800-981-5721

Rhode Island
State Hotline   1-800-726-3010
                 401-831-5522

AIDS Care Ocean State
401-521-3603   (Providence)
www.aidscareos.org

Planned Parenthood Rhode Island Clinic
401-421-9620   (Providence)

Urban League of Rhode Island
401-351-5000   (Providence)
www.ulri.org

South Carolina
State Hotline   1-800-322-2437
                803-898-0749

Beaufort County Health Department
843-757-2251   (Bluffton)

Columbus AIDS Task Force
614-299-2437   (Columbus)

Low Country AIDS Services
843-747-2273   (North Charleston)

South Carolina African American
HIV/AIDS Council
803-254-6644   (Columbia)
www.scaahac.org

The Access Network
843-681-2437   (Hilton Head)

The Citadel
843-953-5230   (Charleston)

South Dakota
State Hotline   1-800-592-1861
                605-773-3737

Berakha House
605-332-4017   (Sioux Falls)

Planned Parenthood of Minnesota
605-361-5100   (Sioux Falls)
South Dakota Department of Health
605-773-3361   (Pierre)

Tennessee
State Hotline   1-800-525-AIDS
                615-741-7500
First Response Center
615-251-6128   (Nashville)
www.metropolitanfrc.com

Friends for Life AIDS Resource Ctr.
901-272-0855   (Memphis)
www.friendsforlifecorp.org

Kids on the Block of Middle Tennessee
615-333-6356   (Nashville)
www.kltb.org

Metropolitan Interdenominational
 Church
615-726-3876   (Nashville)
www.metopolitainfrc.com

Minority AIDS Outreach
615-391-3737   (Nashville)

Nashville Cares
615-259-4866   (Nashville)
www.nashvillecares.org

New Directions Inc.
901-327-4244   (Memphis)
newdirtn@bellsouth.net

Planned Parenthood
901-725-1717   (Memphis)

Tennessee Department of Health
615-741-3111   (Memphis)
www.state.tn.us/health

Texas
State Hotline   1-800-299-2437
                512-490-2505

AIDS Foundation of Houston
713-623-6796   (Houston)
www.aidshelp.org

AIDS Interfaith Network (AIN)
214-941-7696 (Dallas)
www.aidsinterfaithnetwork.org

AIDS Interfaith Network (AIN)
817-870-4800 (Fort Worth)
www.adsinterfaithnetwork.org

AIDS Outreach Center
817-335-1994 (Fort Worth)
www.alc.org

AIDS Resource Center
214-521-5124 (Dallas)
www.resourcecenterdallas.org

AIDS Services of Austin
512-458-2437 (Austin)
www.asaustin.org

Austin Outreach and Community
512-833-0444 (Austin)

Block Effort Against the Threat of
AIDS (BEAT)
210-212-2266 (San Antonio)

Body Positive Houston
713-830-3033 (Houston)
www.montroseclinic.org

Bread of Life Inc.
713-650-0595 (Houston)

Cascade AIDS Project
503-223-5907 (Portland)
www.cascadeaids.org

Crisis Intervention Hotline
713-527-9864 (Houston)
www.crisishotline.org

Coastal Bend AIDS Foundation
361-814-2001 (Corpus Christi)

Dallas Urban League
214-915-4600 (Dallas)

Families Under Urban and Social Attack
713-651-1470 (Houston)
www.fuusa.org

HIV Outreach Prevention Education
Project (HOPE)
713-674-0231 (Houston)
www.africanvillage.com

Hope Action Care (HAC)
210-224-7330 (San Antonio)

Human Services Network Inc.
214-330-5130 (Dallas)

Lasima Foundation
214-941-1132 (Dallas)
www.lasima.org

Lifeworks
512-441-8336 (Austin)
www.lifeworksweb.org

NAACP
713-526 -3389 (Houston)
www.naacphouston.org

Out Youth Austin
512-419-1233 (Austin)
www.outyouth.org

Planned Parenthood of Dallas and
Northeast Texas
214-363-2004 (Dallas)

Renaissance III Inc.
214-421-4343 (Dallas)
www.renaissance3.com

San Antonio AIDS Foundation
210-225-4715 (San Antonio)

Texas AIDS Network
512-447-8887 (Austin)
ten@global.org

Texas Department of Health

512-458-7111   (Austin)

The Center for AIDS
713-527-8219   (Houston)
www.centerforaids.org

University of Texas Southwestern
Medical Center
214-645-7300 or 944-1050   (Dallas)
www.2.utsouthwestern.edu.cpiu

WAM Foundation, Inc.
713-551-8787   (Houston)
wam@foundation.org

Utah

State Hotline   1-800-366-2437
                801-366-2437

People with AIDS Coalition of Utah
801-484-2205   (Salt Lake City)

Planned Parenthood
801-322-1586   (Salt Lake City)

Utah Department of Health
801-538-6111   (Salt Lake City)
www.health.state.ut.us/els/hivaids

Vermont

State Hotline   1-800-882-2437
                802-863-7245

Hilltop Light Ministries
802-863-0524   (Burlington)
www.hilltop.org

Vermont Cares
802-863-2437   (Burlington)
www.vtcares.org

Vermont Department of Health
802-863-7200   (Burlington)

Virginia

State Hotline   1-800-533-4148

Alternative House
703-356-6360   (Dun Loring)
www.thealternativhealth.org

Central Virginia HIV Care
Consortium
804-828-8844   (Richmond)
www.views.vcu.edu/hiv

Northern Virginia AIDS Ministry
703-746-0440   (Arlington)
www.novam.org

Richmond AIDS Consortium
804-828-6471   (Richmond)
www.cpcra.org

Tidewater AIDS Crisis TaskForce
757-583-1317   (Norfolk)
www.tact-online.com

Washington

State Hotline   1-800-272-2437
                360-236-3466
Babes Network
206-720-5566   (Seattle)
www.babesnetwork.org

Cascade AIDS Project
503-223-5907   (Vancouver)
www.cascadeaids.org

People of Color Against AIDS
Network
1-877-POCAAN-9   Main Number
1-205-322-7061   POCAAN Seattle
1-253-272-2577   POCAANTacoma
1-509-249-8725   POCAAN Yakima

Seattle Couseling Service
206-323-1768   (Seattle)
www.seattlecounseling.org

Shanti Multifaith Works
206-324-1520   (Seattle)
www.multifaith.org

Spokane Aids Network
509-455-8993   (Spokane)
www.spokanaidsnetwork.org

Youth Care Adolescent Health
206-694-4500   (Seattle)

University of Washington (FHCRC)
206-667-2300   (Seattle)
www.washington.edu

West Virginia
State Hotline   1-800-642-8244
                304-558-2950

Charleston AIDS Network
304-345-4673   (Charleston)
www.aidsnet.net

West Virginia Department of Health
304-558-2950   (Charleston)
www.wvdhhr.org

Wisconsin
State Hotline   1-800-991-5533
                414-273-2437

AIDS Resource Center of Wisconsin
262-657-6644   (Kenosha)

AIDS Resource Center of Wisconsin
920-437-7400   (Green Bay)

AIDS Resource Center of Wisconsin
414-273-1991   (Milwaukee)
www.arcw.org

Black Health Coalition of Wisconsin
414-933-0064   (Milwaukee)
www.blackhealthcoalition.com

Center for Child and Family Services
414-442-4702   (Milwaukee)

16th Street Community Health Center
414-672-1353   (Milwaukee)
www.sschc.org

Wyoming
State Hotline   1-800-327-3577

Sheridan County Community Health
206-672-9791   (Sheridan)

United Medical Center West
307-634-2273   (Sheridan)
www.umccwy.info)

OTHER HELPFUL WEBSITES

www.advocatesforyouth.org
202-419-3420   (Washington, DC)

Africa Peace Education Program
APEPS HIV/AIDS Inititives
404-586-0460   (Atlanta, GA)
www.afsc.org/agep/aids

Hip Hop Summit Action Network
(HSAN) Taking Back Responsibility
www.hiphopsummitactionnetwork.org

www.hivandhepatitis.com

www.ourbodyourselves.org

The Tavis Smiley Foundation
323-290-1888   (Los Angeles, CA)
www.tavistalks.com

The HIV/AIDS Authority
www.thebody.com

US AID Health: HIV/AIDS
202-712-4320   (Washington, DC)
www.usaid.gov

Bibliography

Afua, Queen, *Sacred Woman: A Guide to Healing the Feminine Body, Mind and Spirit,* New York, NY.: One World Ballantine Books, 2000

AIDS Info NYC Organization, *HIV + Issue 10: To tell the Truth,* www.aidsinfonyc.org, October 2000

Akbar, Na'Im, *Know Thy Self,* Tallahassee, FL.: Mind Productions & Associates, 1998

American Social Health Association, *Facts & Answers about STD's: Introduction to Sexually Transmitted Diseases (STD's),* www.ashastd.org, 2001

American Social Health Association, Booklet, *For Teens: Some Questions and Answers about STD's for Teens,* 1998

Avert, *AIDS Education & Young People at School,* www.avert.com, May 1999

Avert, *Using Condoms, Condom Types and Condom Sizes,* www.avert.com, November 2001

Badiner, Allan Hunt, *(Editor), Mindfulness in the Marketplace: Compassionate Responses to Consumerism,* Berkeley, CA.: Parallax Press, 2002

Balm of Gilead, New York, NY.: www.thebalmingilead.org, 2003

Brower, Jennifer and Chalk, Peter, *The Global Threat of New and Reemerging Infectious Diseases, Reconciling U.S. National Security and Public Health Policy,* Santa Monica, CA.: Rand, 2003

Centers for Disease Control and Prevention (CDC), Booklet, *Be a Force for Change: Talk with Young People About HIV,* 2000

Centers for Disease Control and Prevention (CDC), *Division of HIV/ AIDS Prevention, What Are Rapid HIV Tests,* www.cdc.gov, 2003

Centers for Disease Control and Prevention (CDC), *Fact Sheet, HIV/ AIDS Among African Americans,* www.cdc.gov/hiv/pubs/facts, 2002

Centers for Disease Control and Prevention (CDC), *Fact Sheet, Need for Sustained HIV Prevention Among Men Who Have Sex with Men,* www.cdc.gov/hiv/pubs/facts, 2001

Centers for Disease Control and prevention (CDC), *HIV/AIDS Surveillance Report, 2002;* Volume 14 (No. 1)

D.A.R.E., (Drug Abuse Resistance Education) Drug Information, www.dare.com, 2002

Diallo, Yaya and Hall, Mitchell, *The Healing Drum: African Wisdom Teachings,* Rochester VT.: Destiny Books, 1989

Franklin, A.J. and Nancy Boyd, *Boys Into Men: Raising Our African American Teenage Sons,* New York, NY.: Dutton, 2000

Gilbert, Steve, *The Tattoo Book,* New York, NY.: Juno Books, 2001

Hanh, Tich Nhat, *The Miracle of Mindfulness: An Introduction to the Practice of Meditation,* Boston, MA.: Beacon Press, 1975

Healthwise Inc., Web MD Corporation, Boise, Idaho, 1996-2003

Heart to Heart Talk with Phillip S. Chua, M.D., *Hepatitis: The Silent Killer, CEBU Cardo Vascular Center,* www.cdc.-cdh.edu/hospial/cardio

HIV/AIDS Resources: *A National Directory,* 8th. Edition, Longmont, CA.: Guides for Living, 2002

Kabat Zinn, Jon, *Mindfulness Meditation,* Chicago, IL.: Nightingale-Conant Corporation, 2002

Kujisource, *HIV: Grave Challenge Faces Young People. Parents: Especially Black,* Los Angeles, CA.: www.blackaids.org, June 2002

Kunjufu, Jawanza, *To Be Popular or Smart: The Black Peer Group.*

Chicago, IL.: African American Images, 1988

Michigan HIV News: Teen News National, *More Adolescents Abstaining from Sex and More Teens Dissatisfied with Sex Education Classes,* www.mihivnews.com, February 4, 2002

Mitchem, Tameka, *Shethang Profile – Hydeia Broadbent,* www.harlemlive.org, September 2000

National Institute of AIDS, *Division of Microbiology & Infectious Diseases: What You Should Know About Hepatitis C,* www.niaid.nih.gov/dmin/hepatitis, 2001

Neimark, Philip John, *The Way of the Orisa: Empowering Your life Through the Ancient African Religion of Ife,* New York, NY.: Harper Collins, 1993

New York Times, *A New Generation: Teenagers Living with H.I.V.,* www.nytimes.com, November 20, 2001

NPR Programming, *Remembering Tuskegee: Syphilis Study Still Provokes Disbelief, Sadness,* www.npr.org/programs, July 2002

Ofori-Ansa, Kwaku, Chart: *Meanings of Symbols in Adinkra Cloth,* Hyattsville, MD.: Sankofa Edu-Cultural Publications, 2000

Planned Parenthood Federation of America Inc., *Birth Control: The Condom,* www.plannedparenthood.org, 2003

Planned Parenthood, Booklet, *The Facts of Life: A Guide for Teens and Their Families,* 1999

Some', Malidoma Patrice, *The Healing Wisdom of Africa: Finding Life Purpose Through Nature, Ritual and Community,* New York, NY.: Jeremy P. Tarcher/Putnam, 1998

Stewart, Julia, *African Proverbs and Wisdom: A Collection for Every Day of the Year, From More Than Forty African Nations,* New York, NY.: Kensington Publishing Corporation, 1997

The Body, *CDC/News Updates: Hydeia Broadbent, 17 Has AIDS But it Doesn't Define Her,* www.thebody.com, December 2001

The California Buddhist Society, *Mindfulness: The Characteristics of Mindfulness (Sati),* www.dharma.ncf.ca/introduction/instructions/sati

U.S. National Library of Medicine and the National Institutes of Health, *Medline Plus Health Information, One in Five U.S. Teens Have Sex Before Age 15,* www.nlm.nih.gov/medlineplus, 2003

U.S. National Library of Medicine and the National Institutes of Health, *Medline Plus Health Information, Tattoos Source of Hepatitis with Symptoms: Study,* www.nlm.nih.gov/medlineplus, 2003

Vanzant, Iyanla, *Act of Faith: Daily Meditations for People of Color,* New York, NY.: Simon and Shuster, 1995

Vanzant, Iyanla, *The Value In The Valley: A Black Woman's Guide Through Life's Dilemmas,* New York, NY.: Simon and Shuster, 1995

Willis, W. Bruce, *The Adinkra Dictionary: A Visual Primer of the Language of Adinkra,* Washington, D.C.: The Pyramid Complex, 1988

Worldwide Online Meditation Center, *Mindfulness Meditation,* Meditation Center, www.meditationcenter.com, 1998-2000

Zingale, Dan, Booklet, *AIDS Action:Talking About AIDS So America Listens,* Washington D.C.: Gil Foundation

ABOUT THE AUTHOR

Deborah Day is a poet, author, mentor, publisher, activist and business consultant. She was born and raised in a small town in the Midwest. Her path led her to Chicago where she lived for 17 years. After graduating from DePaul University, she worked for several major corporations in sales and marketing. In 1994 she and her son relocated to California's Bay Area. In 1997 she started her own business Ashay by the Bay.

She wrote and self published, **Mindful Messages** *Healing Thoughts for the Hip and Hop Descendants from the Motherland.* When she learned that African Americans were 50% of the newly reported HIV/AIDS cases she decided to refocus her efforts of another nearly completed book to address HIV/AIDS Awareness and Prevention for youth. She advocates abstinence first and supports safe sex for those who are sexually active. After completing the book she created the **Mindful Messages Mentoring Program** and wrote the curriculum for the workbook. This program is designed to educate youth about their culture and history and to empower them with HIV/AIDS Awareness and Prevention and life-skills information. With both the book and workbook, parents can mentor their children at home. The Mindful Messages Mentoring Program also easily adapts to a classroom environment as a tool for educators.

Her poet name is Ashay (sometimes spelled Ashe) and means "spirituality and life force" it is also spoken to acknowledge and honor our ancestors. Her poetic style is alliteration but she is experimenting with other creative forms. In 2003, she was named the Readers and Writers Advantage Author of the Year. She is a member of the San Francisco Bay Book Writers Guild, HIV Prevention Planning Council (HPPC) and The African American HIV/AIDS Task Force. Currently she is promoting the Mindful Messages Mentoring Program and working with youth.

Mindful Notes

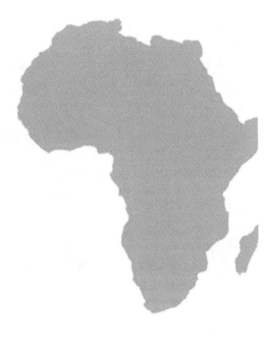

Mindful Notes

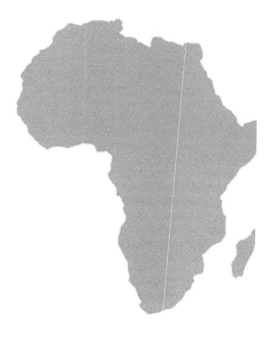

Mindful Notes

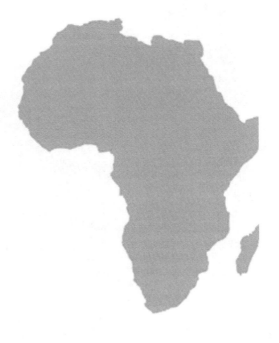

Mindful Notes

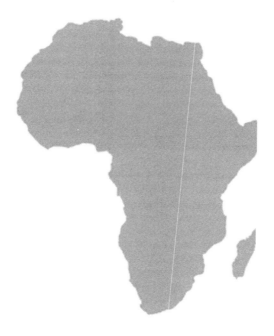

Mindful Notes

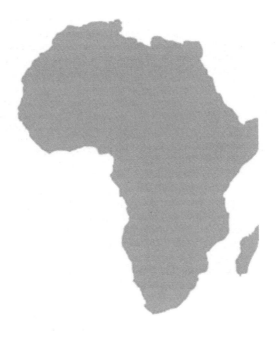

Yes, I want to reorder **Mindful Messages**

Mindful Messages Mentoring is great for one on one at home mentoring or in the classroom!

Mindful Messages teaches African American youth ages 12-19 about HIV/AIDS Awareness and Prevention education from an Africentric perspective. Mindful Messages creatively builds character while it increases cultural awareness, self-awareness and self-esteem. Purchase the book and workbook and become a Mindful Messenger through the Mindful Messages Mentoring Program.

Mindful Messages contains: 26 Spoken Word poems, African proverbs, information on Mindfulness Meditation, HIV/AIDS, STD's, Drugs, Peer Pressure, Abstinence, Safe Sex, Relationships, stories of Africans and African Americans Living with HIV/AIDS, The My Choice to Stay Abstinent and Drug Free Agreements, The Adinkra symbols, a National HIV/AIDS resource list, art illustrations and much more. Description: Bright Glossy Cover, Size 5 1/2 x 8 1/2, 192 pages

Mindful Messages Mentoring Workbook contains: 175 Exercises and 45 Mindful Notes formatted within 12 lessons, a map of Africa, graphic art illustrations, African proverbs. (Curriculum is based on the poetic phrases in the Mindful Messages book) Description: Bright Glossy Cover Size 8 1/2 x 11, approx. 46 pages

Date_____

Name_____

Organization_____

Address_____

City_____ State_____ Zip_____

Phone Number _____Fax _____

Email Address:_____

	Qty.	Price	Total
Mindful Messages Book ISBN# 0970404824	_____	14.95	_____
M M Mentoring Workbook ISBN# 0970404832	_____	11.95	
		Subtotal	_____
Shipping and Handling Charges California Residents Tax(8.25%)			_____
$3.00/book $2.00/workbook			
*Volume Discounts Available		Shipping & Handling	_____

Method of Payment   Total $ _____

Check #_____ Credit Card: Visa or Mastercard # _____

Expiration Date _____

Name on Card _____

Place your order by mail, phone, fax or directly from our website.
Ashay by the Bay   P. O. Box 2394   Union City, California 94587
Phone: 510-520-2742   Fax: 510-477-0967   Website: www.ashaybythebay.com